Politics and the Expanding Physician Supply

OTHER VOLUMES IN THE

Conservation of Human Resources Series

COMPARATIVE METROPOLITAN EMLOYMENT COMPLEXES: NEW YORK, CHICAGO, LOS ANGELES, HOUSTON AND ATLANTA (7)
Dale L. Hiestand and Dean W. Morse

COLLECTIVE BARGAINING AND MANPOWER UTILIZATION IN BIG CITY GOVERNMENTS (6)
David Lewin, Raymond D. Horton and James W. Kuhn

CONTROLLING SOCIAL EXPENDITURES: THE SEARCH FOR OUTPUT MEASURES (8)
Alfred S. Eichner and Charles Brecher

SUBURBANIZATION AND THE CITY (2)
Thomas M. Stanback, Jr. and Richard V. Knight

LABOR MARKETS: SEGMENTS AND SHELTERS (1)
Marcia Freedman with Gretchen Maclachlan

HEALTH MANPOWER AND HEALTH POLICY (10)
Eli Ginzberg

EARLY RETIREMENT: BOON OR BANE? (14)
Dean Morse and Susan H. Gray

WOMEN RETURNING TO WORK: POLICIES AND PROGRESS IN FIVE COUNTRIES (12)
Alice M. Yohalem

THE CAREERS OF PROFESSIONAL WOMEN: COMMITMENT AND CONFLICT (5)
Alice Yohalem

PRIDE AGAINST PREJUDICE: WORK IN THE LIVES OF OLDER BLACKS AND YOUNG PUERTO RICANS (9)
Dean W. Morse

BRIDGES TO WORK: INTERNATIONAL COMPARISONS OF TRANSITION SERVICES (3)
Beatrice G. Reubens

Politics and the Expanding Physician Supply

by **MICHAEL L. MILLMAN**

Foreword by Eli Ginzberg

LANDMARK STUDIES
Allanheld Osmun MONTCLAIR
Universe Books NEW YORK

Allanheld, Osmun & Co. Publishers, Inc.
19 Brunswick Road, Montclair, N.J. 07042

Published in the United States of America in 1980
by Allanheld, Osmun & Co. and by Universe Books
381 Park Avenue South, New York, N.Y. 10016
Distribution: Universe Books

LIBRARY OF CONGRESS CATALOGING IN PUBLICATION DATA

Millman, Michael L
Politics and the expanding physician supply.

(Conservation of human resources series; 11)
(Landmark studies)
Bibliography: p.
Includes index.
1. Medical education policy—United States.
2. Medical education policy—Illinois. 3. Physicians—United States—Supply and demand. I. Title. II. Series.
R745.M615 610'.8'1173 78-73591
ISBN 0-87663-841-8

Printed in the United States of America

To the memory of my father
Joseph Millman

Contents

TABLES AND FIGURES

Tables

Figure

Foreword

The word has gone out from Washington that something is seriously wrong with the nation's health manpower, particularly its physician manpower. In place of the long-touted shortages that dominated public discussion and action in the 1960s, we now are told of the dangers which the nation faces from the coming oversupply of physicians, each one of whom, it is estimated, may add one-quarter of a million dollars to our annual health expenditures.

This book does not deal primarily with the forces that led to the widespread acceptance of the shortage theorem and that more recently have warned of an approaching surplus. Rather, Dr. Millman has focused his analysis upon the structural relations among the federal government, state governments, and the medical institutions as public policy moved with increasing vigor to expand the supply of physician manpower. His is a study of intergovernmental relations, more specifically "private federalism," a term which he uses to describe the interaction between the federal government and the principal medical institutions cooperating to increase the supply of physicians. At the same time that the federal government moved directly and forcefully to accomplish new national goals respecting the supply of physicians in general and certain specialties in particular, principally family practice, it paid little attention to the actions or reactions of state governments that historically have been involved in planning, financing and operating a significant proportion of the nation's medical schools.

At first glance it is difficult to understand how our federal-state system could have been relegated to the sidelines while the federal government, with the bit in its mouth, undertook to deal directly with the medical establishment with scarcely a nod in the direction of state governments. But state governments, with only a few exceptions, were also impelled by the same problem—the shortage of physicians—to heroic remedial efforts, notably a substantial increase in their allocations for the support of medical education.

One of the important questions that the reader should ask himself as he reads this interesting and illuminating account about the parallel actions of the federal and state governments is whether a more carefully coordinated effort between these two levels of governments would have resulted in significantly different outcomes either in terms of the objectives pursued or how well they were achieved. I, for one, seriously question whether a deliberate and continuous effort on the part of the federal government to work closely with state governments would have had any effect other than to slow the process of expansion, not because a slower rate of expansion was desired or necessarily desirable but solely because of the difficulties of achieving coordination.

The other principal dimension of Millman's inquiry is to lay bare the important interactions between the medical establishment and the federal government to speed the expansion, once the medical leadership reached consensus that such an expansion was in the public's and their own interest. A careful reading of Dr. Millman's richly detailed reconstruction is a potent reminder of how difficult it has been—and probably will continue to be—for even the federal government to move strongly in the pursuit of any service goal without the active support and cooperation of the key private interest groups. In the case of medical education, these include the publicly-supported medical schools.

Federal initiative and federal dollars can bring about important changes in the structure of such conservative institutions as medical schools but whether such changes as reflected in enlarged enrollments, the increasing percentage of low income and minority group students, the expansion of residency training in family practice will accomplish the ends that Congress seeks—improved health care for underserved populations in the inner city and in rural areas—remains moot. I believe I read Millman correctly as warning not to overestimate the influence of the Congress to alter the practice of medicine, unless it goes much further than it has yet been willing to go to erode the power of both the states and the medical establishment. Reformulated, the important lesson that can be extracted from Millman is that a more carefully planned and executed effort to control the number of physicians, their specialties, and their practice locations would require preemption by the federal government of powers long in the domain of the states and at the same time a major contraction in the powers that have been exercised by organized medicine and individual providers of service.

If this is in fact one correct deduction from Millman's perceptive analysis, another could be formulated thus: how far can our society go to alter the patterns of output and distribution of physicians if it is unwilling to sacrifice more seriously the long-term pluralistic division of powers? Clearly the federal government can go a fair distance in altering its financial support for the training of health professionals although it remains to be seen whether, in the face of the precarious position of many medical schools, it will be able to eliminate capitation payments. It is more likely to be able to terminate funds for expansion. The probability of effecting a radical reduction in the inflow of foreign medical graduates given the dependence of selected states on this source of manpower is uncertain. Even more problematic is the ability of the federal government to affect the distribution of physicians by specialty or by location. One need not argue that the federal government has no cards to play but only that the other players—state governments and the medical establishment—also have strong hands. Present planning in Washington includes such diverse approaches as monetary incentives, fee controls, loans with paybacks in the form of service, changes in reimbursement practices, national licensing, certifications involving the right to establish a practice in specified areas and still other tried and untried measures. The important point to remember in reading Millman's account of private federalism is the non-symmetry between efforts to expand physician supply which all parties perceived to be advantageous—medical schools, hospitals and the community—and efforts to alter the characteristics of the supply, particularly its distribution, which to date remain more theory than accomplishment.

Since I have taken liberties in sharing with the reader what I have inferred from Millman's analysis, I will take one more step down that road to make explicit the underlying lesson that I have found in his cautionary tale. It is this.

There is no possible way in a democratic country of continental proportions such as the United States to accomplish rapid changes in the delivery of any complex service through action by the federal government alone. All one need do to confirm this generalization is to be reminded that postal services are the only direct service the federal government provides to the American people. Everything else, from employment services to education, is either shared with the states and localities or is in the exclusive domain of these lower levels of government. The matter is even more complicated in the case of medical services where major nonprofit institutions such as hospitals and the Blues play a critical role and where most physicians are still in the private practice of medicine. Given predominant roles of state and local governments, the importance of nonprofit institutions and the continuing scope for initiative by the private sector, the federal government must moderate its interventions accordingly. This is not to say that it can only stand on the sidelines and eschew all action aimed at rationalizing to some degree its large-scale investments in health manpower to insure that they add rather than subtract to the effectiveness and efficiency of health services delivery. But the key words are "to some degree." The federal government has no option but to set its goals and to pursue them at a pace determined by its success in prevailing upon other levels of government, particularly the states, and the nonprofit and profit sectors, to join it in pursuing the same goals through parallel and complementary approaches.

Not every reader may extract this lesson from Millman's work but it is the one that impressed me. It may prove a stimulating introduction to those who are yet to study this insightful account of private federalism in the 1960s-early 1970s, a time when the federal government undertook to expand the supply of physician manpower.

Eli Ginzberg, Director
Conservation of Human Resources
Columbia University
June 1979

Acknowledgments

This volume is based on a dissertation funded by a grant from The Robert Wood Johnson Foundation to the Conservation of Human Resources Project, Columbia University. I would like to thank the Foundation and Dr. Eli Ginzberg for furnishing the financial support and working environment without which this study could not have been completed.

I am grateful to Dr. Bruce Smith of the Columbia University Political Science Department, not only for his sponsorship of the dissertation, but his unflagging interest and continuing guidance throughout my career at Columbia.

I would also like to express my gratitude to the Conservation of Human Resources staff. Throughout all stages of this study, Dr. Eli Ginzberg provided valuable direction and incisive editorial advice. I am especially indebted to Miriam Ostow and Charles Brecher, who were always available when I needed counsel and a critical eye.

The Illinois case study would have suffered immeasurably without the support and interest of Dr. Donald Caseley of the University of Illinois. The following individuals were kind enough to allow me to intrude upon their busy schedules for information about the Illinois medical education scene: James McGill, James Campbell, Mark Lepper, Robert Hendrickson, and David Knoll.

I would further wish to acknowledge the many friends and colleagues who made the task of writing this dissertation easier. In particular, I would like to mention Phyllis Endreny, Patricia McFate, and Corinne Kirchner for their time and comments.

1

Introduction

Growing recognition of the blurred distinction between private and public sector activities in the United States has generated an increased sensitivity to a new dimension of governmental decision-making. Murray Weidenbaum in *The Modern Public Sector* argues that choices between specific program-areas—whether to put additional funds into education versus health, for instance—are not the only choices to be made:

> Basic aspects of governmental decisions now involve selecting the mechanism through which the government will act to achieve its objectives. The question is no longer, "which government agency should be assigned the new program?" Rather, the problem has been broadened to include such options as setting up new federal agencies or drawing on existing expertise outside of the federal government. If the latter route is chosen, another set of questions then comes to the fore: "Should the states be involved, via grants-in-aid?" or "Should private industry be assigned to the actual administration through business contracts negotiated between the corporation and the government?"[1]

The choices are complex and the decisions may be momentous. To assess them is a challenge. What follows is a report of a study that undertook that challenge. Specifically, this study assesses the mechanism by which government in recent years has sought to ensure an adequate supply of physicians for the nation.

The first observation to make about medical education is the most basic: Public sector authority in this arena is divided among the federal government and several states. Thereafter the picture becomes complicated, because private groups as well have been delegated responsibility to exercise quasi-governmental authority. In order to understand the governance of the physician production process, one needs to understand the rather complex patterns of interaction among these actors.

Since 1963, Congress has enacted several pieces of legislation that have significantly increased the federal government's role in the production of physicians. States, however, have traditionally supported public medical schools and, in some cases, even have provided subsidies to private schools within their borders. Between 1965 and 1975 the federal government spent $1.6 billion on aid to medical education,[2] while states now spend $.5 billion *annually* for general medical school operating support.[3]

When the federal government assumes additional responsibilities in social policy, there is often considerable controversy over whether state and local governments will wither away under the impact of federal influence. The national grants-in-aid system, for example, has provided fertile ground for the study of federal control at the state and local levels. Researchers in health policy have worried over intergovernmental problems associated with Medicaid,[4] the establishment of community mental health centers,[5] and federal child health programs.[6] The intergovernmental perspective, however, has been almost totally lacking from health manpower policy analysis.

Why this omission? A major reason is that federal aid to medical education does not follow the traditional, easily recognizable intergovernmental pattern. In Medicaid, community mental health centers, the Hill-Burton hospital construction program, Comprehensive Health Planning, and similar programs, the federal government required direct state-local involvement through such devices as mandatory planning activities, state matching funds, and the establishment of state-local standards. All of these mechanisms required direct communication among the various levels of government. Indeed, the history of health and other social legislation in the 1960s and 1970s involves the search for ways to strengthen state and local management of federal programs. While this search has been slowed by lapses of confidence in the capability of state and local governments, a vigorous debate has always existed over how the various levels of government should relate to one another. The ideal of "partnership" has been celebrated in rhetoric, but it has been elusive in practice.

Federal health manpower programs resemble biomedical and other types of research funding and deal, for the most part, directly with institutions—namely, medical schools—that receive aid. This mode of governmental operation has been variously called "private federalism" or "federalism by contract." However named, the concept has been delineated well; surprisingly, only the beginnings of significant research efforts are discernible.

Daniel Elazar defines private federalism as "the extension of federal aid to individuals, public nongovernmental bodies, or even profit-making concerns to perform specific public services." He notes that universities have been the primary recipients of such aid for campus construction and student support, as well as for research and demonstration projects. "In the former case," says Elazar, "since the federal government has required that private as well as public universities be subject to state higher education planning, these grants have become, willy-nilly, integrated into the state system to provide an often unrecognized extra measure of federal aid to the states." He further suggests that private federalism "contains potential dangers to the states' ability to control governmental activities within their boundaries."[7]

Outside the stream of literature, whose express purpose is to explore the nature of federalism, is another source. The term "federalism by contract" devolves from the latter. In 1954, Don K. Price suggested that scientists engaged in research and development has helped to promote "an improvised system of federalism that makes use of private institutions for the conduct of federal programs."[8] Bruce Smith points out that it is not the idea of the federal government contracting for services that is new. After all, from the earliest days of the republic, government contracted for building roads and delivering mail. What *is* new is the magnitude of government contracting for rather esoteric services. Here one begins to perceive the critical tension between *accountability* and *independence*—"the line which separates legitimate oversight from excessive and self-defeating intrusion into the contractor's internal management."[9]

The two bodies of work associated respectively with "private federalism" and with "federalism by contract" raise interesting issues for analysis of the medical education sector. The incontrovertible fact is that states have had a traditional, substantial, and continuing role in medical education, in contrast to policy areas of defense or scientific research, and this underscores the importance of examining the relationship among levels of government following a large new federal input, i.e., private federalism. In view of the role of professional groups and private institutions that receive little state support, it is also relevant to discuss matters of independence and accountability usually associated with "federalism by contract." For convenience, however, I will use the term "private federalism" throughout this study.

Federal policy-makers chose the route of private federalism to expand the supply of physicians. Alternatively, they might have allocated money to the states to be distributed to the medical schools: They could have required the states to submit plans for increasing their physician supply, or they might have mandated state contributions for medical school construction. Indeed, as we shall see, such proposals were offered but largely ignored.

In reality, the federal decision was to bypass the states—to use private federalism in favor of normal intergovernmental transfers. This policy reflected not so much a choice between alternative policies as it did the political and structural characteristics of health manpower as a policy arena and also the historical relationship of medical schools to government. Much of this study will be devoted to describing and analyzing those characteristics to understand better why this nation went about expanding its physician supply in the way it did. Since private federalism is a major mechanism of disbursing public funds for health resources, it is essential that we understand how it operates, the results it produces, and the problems it creates.

In essence, this is a study of government's attempts to intervene in a complex social process—the production and deployment of physicians. The process is dominated by powerful interest groups and multifaceted institutions.

INTERGOVERNMENTAL RELATIONS, PRIVATE FEDERALISM, AND HEALTH POLICY

An essential feature of American government is its federal structure. "There is little about government that is more important than the interrelationships between the several levels and units through which it operates," writes W. Brooke Graves. "How well these units are working together at any given time, in their day-to-day operations, almost provides an index to how well government as a whole is functioning."[10]

All levels of government in the United States have significantly participated in efforts to expand and shape the physician supply through the financing and planning of medical education. Students of intergovernmental relations should have little difficulty accepting this notion of shared powers in the area of health manpower policy. They need only refer to Morton Grodzins, who said, in his pioneering work on modern federalism: "All levels of government in the United States significantly participate in all activities of government."[11] This is a deceptively simple point of view. Commenting on its importance, Elazar observed of Grodzins: "He clearly recognized that federalism—at least in an age of complexity and interdependence such as ours—was not a matter of isolating governments for separate (and minimal) action but of sharing powers for interdependent accomplishment."[12]

Nevertheless, there is a disturbing lack of appreciation of the concept of shared powers for interdependent accomplishment. Consider the recommendations for state and federal responsibilities often prescribed by public and private commissions that have addressed the issue of physician supply. Among them: "There should be greater emphasis on federal-state cooperation in overcoming geographic maldistribution;[13] an independent national coordinating agency on medical manpower supported by private foundations should be created;[14] the federal government should provide stable, long-term support for medical schools because they are "national resources."[15] All such recommendations seemingly have been made without a full understanding of the political realities of their implementation.

What past and present political relationships ought to be taken into account in the process of formulating future policies? When that question is put, we see that there are some important gaps in our knowledge. Thus it is relevant to ask: What barriers stand in the way of federal-state cooperation and what mechanisms will facilitate cooperation? What is the likelihood that an independent, coordinating body will succeed in light of older, well-established patterns of political behavior? Given past federal legislative, administrative, and budgetary politics, what conditions must obtain before a stable base of support for the training of highly paid professionals can be maintained?

Policy-makers cannot begin to answer these questions until they have a better understanding of two prior issues. *First,* what functions does each level of government perform in the medical education sector, and how do these functions relate to other policy areas? *Second,* how do the levels of government relate to one another? It is the central task of this study to shed light on these two areas.

The general approach taken by others to intergovernmental policy and analysis has been primarily to measure the political, administrative, fiscal, and service impacts of federal programs at the state level. Altenstetter and Bjorkman, for example, examined the impact of federal child health programs on the State of Connecticut from three perspectives: (1) the performance of the state in achieving the explicit federal goals of stimulating the provision of direct services; (2) the indirect impact of federal initiatives on the state's administrative capabilities; and (3) the reciprocal effects of state and local influences on federal policy.[16]

A dominant approach in intergovernmental studies is to begin with federal goals as stated in legislation, regulations, and other policy statements and then trace their implementation or frustration at the state-local level. Of key interest have been "vertical functional autocracies," the interlevel linkages between like-minded program specialists or professionals, whose loyalties rest more with their program area than with the level of government they represent. This is said to have created problems with respect to interprogram, interagency, and interprofessional competition, as well as a possible loss of policy control by generalist politicians and appointive officials.[17]

As difficult as it is to measure policy impacts in federal programs that require an explicit state-local role, the problems are compounded when dealing with private federalism. In private federalism, there is no explicit role for states and local governments; therefore one cannot examine implementation of federal objectives through state and local performance in the usual sense. The focus of the assessment of governmental activity shifts to how well nongovernmental institutions have performed. Medical schools were held directly accountable to the federal government for their use of federal money. Nonetheless, in many cases, these schools were also accountable to the state governments. To their advantage as well as disadvantage, schools found themselves between two masters, each with a carrot and a stick.

Since linkages between the federal and state governments are formed indirectly through the medical schools, the identification and examination of an operating vertical functional autocracy in this system becomes a knotty problem. A further complication is that medical education policy at the federal level is made by "health" agencies and congressional committees, while at the state level, higher-education agencies and legislative committees have primary jurisdiction. The interest groups, however, tend to combine both the elements of medicine and education.

The problem of studying private federalism requires that special attention be given to an additional dimension of policy development and implementation. The central questions of intergovernmental relations remain relevant:

1. What is the pattern of intergovernmental relations between the federal and state levels?

2. What problems arise as a result of this pattern?

3. What steps could be taken to make the system operate more effectively?

Over and above these questions, we must be particularly sensitive to the subtle means by which levels of government influence one another through the intermediary of nongovernmental bodies. This demands careful charting of the roles and functioning of major actors in the health manpower policy arena.

In addition to the conceptual adjustments necessary to study private federalism, another important problem is the absence of generally agreed-upon objective criteria for measuring whether a policy is "good" or "bad" in terms of achieving an adequate health manpower supply. While this circumstance is not uncommon in other policy arenas, if there is any agreement in the realm of measuring "need," "demand," and "supply" in relation to physician shortages, it is that our ability to accomplish the task is extremely limited—a "mission impossible," in the words of economist Uwe Reinhardt.[18]

Reinhardt and others have discussed the reasons for past failures in health manpower forecasting and the barriers blocking future success,[19] and I need not duplicate their efforts here. Instead, I wish to convey the futility of applying a numerical supply standard to an evaluation of state and federal policies. This is a policy area where, on one hand, analysts can employ a so-called conservative model of physician requirements—as did a 1975 New York State Regents Task Force—and conclude that the state with one of the most favorable physician/population ratios ought to increase its medical school capacity by about one-third.[20] On the other hand, there are health manpower specialists like Eli Ginzberg who have warned for years that effective economical use of physician manpower may well depend upon maintaining a taut supply and that there are other available means of improving access to health-care services.[21]

Furthermore, any attempt to measure public policy against either of these two standards would be inconclusive at this stage because of the lag time between increased investments in medical education and the settling of the additional physicians into practice. I will therefore pursue another course of analysis: to conduct a thorough-going political analysis, in line with the suggestion of one critic of physician manpower forecasts that we must "learn more about the determinants of requirements and supplies and how past reconciliations between them were accomplished.[22] To the extent that physician requirements can be perceived within a wide range depending on whose expertise is sought, and that physician supply is largely determined by governmental expenditures, a political analysis will provide interesting insights into "past reconciliations" between supply and demand, as well as suggest prospects for the future.

ORGANIZATION OF THE STUDY

Let us conceptualize the health manpower policy arena as a triangular relationship among the medical education sector, the federal government, and state and local government. The direct linkages between levels of government are weak, while those between each level of government and the medical education sector are considerably stronger.

The study will begin with an examination of the medical education sector (Chapter 2). I will explore the educational institutions that produce physicians and the governing structures associated with that process. A key concern will be the role of interest groups in performing quasi-governmental tasks and the growing attention of government to how those tasks are performed.

Chapter 3 begins a discussion of the federal role. Examination of congressional activity, as a main focus of analysis, will help clarify legislative intentions: How did Congress perceive the problems of an inadequate physician supply in terms of the appropriate numbers, types, and geographic distribution of doctors? What legislative solutions to the problems did they pursue? What role, if any, did they perceive for states and local governments?

Analysis of the federal role continues in Chapter 4 with implementation and administrative practice as the central topic. How are congressional intentions translated by the executive into action? Congressional control of administration through appropriations, oversight, and executive reorganization is taken into account. Recognition is also given to the role of President and bureaucracy in influencing legislation.

The major objectives of Chapters 3 and 4 is to document the development over time of a federal role that was largely removed from any sharing of functions with state governments. Chapters 5 and 6 are designed to document what the states and local governments were doing during that period in regard to health manpower policy, and how in fact they reclaimed a role for themselves. What was their view of the federal role, and how did federal activities add to or detract from state initiatives? A detailed case study will be reported of one state's (Illinois) efforts to expand its physician supply (Chapters 5 and 6); Chapter 7 then attempts to generalize from the Illinois experience to other states.

Special attention is paid to the heretofore neglected role of local governments in medical education politics. The final chapter offers some concluding observations about the three-cornered relationship among the medical education sector, the federal government, and state and local government. The discussion of the legacy of private federalism leads, in closing, to a consideration of adaptations that are likely to be required in addressing future policy issues.

A word about the case-study approach as employed here: It is designed to communicate an analytical understanding of (a) the decisional processes involved in the formulation and implementation of policies to expand the physician supply; (b) the political and organizational framework within which those decisions were made; and finally (c) the substantive policy problem itself.[23]

Why has Illinois been chosen for the case study? Illinois provides a useful laboratory for two primary reasons: (1) the number and diverse types of medical education institutions within its borders, and (2) the nature of its physician-supply problems. No state is precisely "typical." What was sought was a state that provides a starting point from which a fuller and differentiated analysis of the state role might proceed. In that respect, this study should be considered essentially exploratory in nature. It is a step in pursuit of a better understanding of how states influence and limit the federal government's ability to devise realistic manpower goals.

Illinois serves as an effective starting point in part because it is a microcosm of the national fervor to increase the supply of physicians. The era of expansion was marked by establishment of both a public and a private medical school, the expansion of existing schools, public support for private institutions, and attempts to innovate in structuring medical education programs to meet the state's health manpower needs. Like many other states, Illinois had the problems of physicians unwilling to locate in rural and ghetto areas, declining numbers of primary-care physicians, unstable financial condition of medical schools, and an influx of foreign medical graduates coupled with the loss of its own medical graduates to more attractive areas of the country. Except for the particular severity of this last problem, Illinois does not represent a unique situation in physician manpower, not even with respect to dimensions of public expenditures, population characteristics, political culture, or resources.

NOTES

1. Murray L. Weidenbaum, *The Modern Public Sector: New Ways of Doing the Government's Business* (New York: Basic Books, 1969), p. 5.

2. U.S. Department of Health, Education, and Welfare, Health Resources Administration, Bureau of Health Manpower, Selected Information on Health Professions Schools, Part II: *BHM Support by Program, PY: 1965–75* (Bethesda, Md.), p. 2.

3. Sylvia I. Etzel and John J. Fauser, comp., "Medical Education in the United States: 1975–1976," *Journal of the American Medical Association*, 27 December 1976, p. 2970.

4. Robert Stevens and Rosemary Stevens, *Welfare Medicine in America: A Case Study of Medicaid* (New York: The Free Press, 1974).

5. Robert H. Connery, et al., *The Politics of Mental Health: Organizing Community Mental Health in Metropolitan Areas* (New York: Columbia University Press, 1968).

6. Christa Altenstetter and James Warner Bjorkman, "The Rediscovery of Federalism: The Impact of Federal Child Health Programs on Connecticut State Health Policy Formation and Service Delivery," in *Public Policy Making in a Federal System*, eds. Charles O. Jones and Robert D. Thomas (Beverly Hills: Sage Publications, 1976), pp. 217–37.

7. Daniel J. Elazar, *American Federalism: A View from the States* (New York: Thomas Y. Crowell Company, 1972), p. 76.

8. Don K. Price, *Government and Science: Their Dynamic Relation in American Democracy* (New York: Oxford University Press, 1954), p. 66.

9. Bruce L. R. Smith, "Accountability and Independence in the Contract State," in *The Dilemma of Accountability in Modern Government: Independence versus Control*, eds. Bruce L. R. Smith and D. C. Hague (New York: MacMillan, 1971), p. 13; see also *The New Political Economy: The Public Use of the Private Sector*, ed. Bruce L. R. Smith (London: MacMillan Press, 1975); Clarence H. Danhof, *Government Contracting and Technological Change* (Washington, D. C.: Brookings Institution, 1968); and Harold Orlans, *Science Policy and the University* (Washington, D.C.: Brookings Institution, 1968).

10. W. Brooke Graves, *American Intergovernmental Relations: Their Origins, Historical Development, and Current Status* (New York: Charles Scribner's Sons, 1964), pp. 3–4.

11. Morton Grodzins, *The American System: A New View of Government in the United States*, ed. Daniel J. Elazar (Chicago: Rand McNally, 1966), p. 13.

12. Ibid., p. v.

13. Carnegie Council on Policy Studies in Higher Education, *Progress and Problems in Medical and Dental Education: Federal Support Versus Federal Control* (San Francisco: Jossey-Bass Publishers, 1976), p. 11.

14. Macy Commission, *Physicians for the Future* (New York: Josiah Macy, Jr., Foundation, 1976), pp. 34–36.

15. U.S. Department of Health, Education, and Welfare, Institute of Medicine, *Costs of Education in the Health Professions*, pts I and II, DHEW Publication, no. (HRA) 74–32, January 1974, p. xv.

16. Altenstetter and Bjorkman, "Rediscovery of Federalism," pp. 218–19.

17. Deil S. Wright, "Intergovernmental Relations: An Analytical Overview," *Annals of the American Academy of Political and Social Science* 416 (November 1974): 14–16.

18. **Uwe E. Reinhardt, "Health Manpower Forecasting,"** ***Manpower for Health Care,*** Institute of Medicine, Washington, D.C., IOM Publication no. 74–003, pp. 19–58.

19. See also Lee Hansen, "An Appraisal of Physician Manpower Projections," *Inquiry* 7 (March 1970): 102–13; Judith R. Lave and Samuel Leinhardt, "Medical Manpower Models: Need, Demand and Supply," *Inquiry* 12 (June 1975): 97–125.

20. New York, Report of the Regents Task Force on Medical School Enrollment and Physician Manpower to the Regents of the University of the State of New York, November 1975.

21. Eli Ginzberg, with Miriam Ostow, *Men, Money, and Medicine* (New York: Columbia University Press, 1969).

22. Hansen, "An Appraisal," p. 111.

23. James W. Fesler, "The Case Method in Political Science," in *Essays on the Case Method in Public Administration*, ed. Edwin Bock (New York: Inter-University Case Program, 1962), p. 70.

2

The Medical Education Sector

The term "medical education sector" is used broadly to refer to the complex institutions and interest groups that have the responsibility in our society for training physicians. The training, or production process, at the minimum requires planning, financing, monitoring, regulating, managing, and institutional cooperation.

Perhaps one of the most confounding aspects of the medical education system in the United States is the absence of a focal point of responsibility in the private sector. The nation's physician supply is greatly dependent on the decisions of 117 medical schools, universities, or teaching hospitals as the potential developers of new medical schools and graduate training programs, specialty societies, and professional associations. These components of the private sector, however, are not autonomous. They are at once influenced by one another as well as by numerous outside forces, such as the actions of government or conditions in the economy at large. The professional training of physicians can broadly be divided into two stages: undergraduate medical education and graduate medical education.

UNDERGRADUATE MEDICAL EDUCATION

Along with the importation of foreign physicians, the most significant means at a society's disposal for increasing the supply of physicians is to encourage existing medical schools to expand their training capacity and/or to establish new schools. However, several interrelated factors have tended to limit expansion, including dollar costs, organized medicine's restrictive stance, and the availability of supporting institutions, especially teaching hospitals.

The Cost Constraint

As a practical matter, the decision to train a larger number of physicians should not be taken lightly. The high cost of medical education relative to other training programs appears to prevail from country to country despite such variable factors as methods of higher-education financing, organization of the health-care system, and economic resources. The reasons cited to explain this difference between professional fields generally include the need for expensive laboratory facilities, the necessity of maintaining a high proportion of faculty to students, the need to pay faculty at a level that somewhat offsets their potential earnings in practice, and the costs of providing clinical experience.

While the actual cost of educating a physician may vary considerably from country to country, and within countries from medical school to medical school, it is sufficiently high in most cases to lead to political controversy, which is generally not found in the production of other types of manpower. In the United States, the high costs have forced the medical education sector to eschew self-sufficiency and reliance upon tuition and general university funds and to seek special support from government. Yet, because the costs have been considerable, no one level of government has been willing to assume complete responsibility. As a consequence, political entanglements have broadened and in turn have affected the structure and operation of the medical education sector.

Concern about the high cost of medical education has spurred several studies that have revealed perhaps more about the underlying processes of medical school operations than about cost structures.[1] Much of the difficulty encountered in determining the cost of medical education stems from the three-part mission of the academic medical center—research, teaching, and patient care—that is often carried out simultaneously. The confusion over assigning costs in the joint production of medical school outputs, however, represents more than a problem in cost accounting. It also reflects some of the basic tensions and the bargaining process endemic to medical schools among the basic scientists, clinicians and those most concerned with patient services.

While some observers recommended that medical students ought to bear a larger portion of the costs of their education considering future returns in personal income, there has been a considerable shift in medical school financing to the extent that where tuition accounted for approximately one-half of total revenues of medical schools in 1926–27,[2] it was less than five percent by 1974-75.[3] As can be seen in Table 2.1, the medical school enterprise is now funded by a diversity of sources for a variety of purposes. The political ramifications of such diversity have taken shape in the following ways: (1) diffusion of decision-making authority within the medical schools; (2) an increase in the number of actors with whom medical school officials must bargain; and (3) deeper involvement in health-care policy developments only indirectly related to medical education.

Table 2.1. Medical School Finances.

Source	*Amount[a] 1974-75*	*Percent Distribution*	
Federal contracts and grants			
For research	$ 612,373	20	
For teaching and training	300,443	10	
For public service	107,709	4	
Recovery of indirect costs	175,586	6	
Subtotal	$1,196,111		40
Nonfederal contracts and grants for restricted programs			
Nonfederal contracts and grants for public service	$270,346	9	
Nongovernment contracts and grants for research	130,878	4	
Nonfederal contracts and grants for teaching and training	67,925	2	
State, city, and county contracts and grants for research	16,543	1	
Recovery of indirect costs on nonfederal contracts and grants	19,407	1	
Subtotal	$505,099		17
Medical school/university activities			
Tuition and fees	$130,168	4	
Professional fee (medical service plan) income	303,028	10	
Income from college services	60,870	2	
Income from endowments	58,618	2	
Other income	112,909	4	
Subtotal	$665,593		22
Other sources of funds			
State appropriations	$ 534,848	18	
State, city, and county grants-in-aid, or subsidies to private schools, or payments via interstate compacts	74,059	3	
Unrestricted gifts	29,582	1	
Subtotal	$ 638,489		22
Total	$3,005,292		

[a]Dollars given in thousands.
Source: "Medical Education in the United States 1975-1976," *Journal of the American Medical Association*, 27 December 1976, Table 36, p. 2969.

It has been recognized for some time that the legacy of increased levels of funding for research via grants to individual faculty members has led to a radically altered decision-making environment in medical schools. The ability of deans to control institutional budgets, marshal resources, and pursue long-range planning was eroded.

With respect to patient care, the effect of the growing importance of income from medical service plans is perhaps less well appreciated. Many medical schools were compelled to expand their patient-care activities in the 1960s in order to accommodate growing numbers of students. At the same time, federal patient-care programs like Medicare and Medicaid provided additional monies to support a larger clinical faculty. It has been observed, however, that this last development led to a decreased reliance on part-time and voluntary faculty, an increase in the ratio of full-time-equivalent faculty positions to the number of students, and increased faculty salaries.[4]

These forces impacted the administrative structure that extends both downward and upward from the dean. One clinical department chairman described the qualties required of him as consisting of "the strength of Bismarck when it comes to representing his department in the dean's office, and the patience of a Kissinger when it comes to straightening out difficulties between his divisions."

> We need to acknowledge that the chairman of a modern department of medicine is nothing more than a micro-dean, and whoever heard of a dean with fewer than six associate deans? Some have as many as 16. Of course, chairmen need to realize their limitations, but, more importantly, the chairman's constituency as well as his administrative superiors need to realize how complex his job has become.[5]

The expansion and differentiation of the medical school faculty has also gone hand in hand with an increase in the number of outside actors with whom medical school personnel must interact. On the biomedical research side, many different federal agencies sponsor research. At a minimum, the granting process requires bargaining on overhead costs and compliance with various guidelines. The linkages between sponsor and grantee, however, can become even more complex when institutions apply for large, multifunction programs, as in the establishment of cancer centers. Such umbrella-type programs can create a complex network of relationships within the institution that extend out to the federal bureaucracy in complex ways.

The enlargement of patient-care responsibilities brought medical school officials in contact with a host of new interest groups, from community planning boards to local practitioners. The political entanglements experienced by medical schools in New York City as they engaged in affiliation agreements with municipal hospitals during the mid-1960s has been documented in several studies.[6] In the 1970s, medical centers were forced to cope within an exposed political environment, the problems escalating with the growth in federal and state roles in personal health care. So, developments in health planning legislation, Medicare and Medicaid reimbursement policies, and hospital cost control are among issues that can significantly impact the finances of the academic health center.

With the targeting of federal money in the 1960s specifically for educational purposes, medical schools established new relationships with the federal bureaucracy and with Congress. New federal funds, often matched by increased state government support, strengthened the hand of deans and other administrative officers in setting institutional policy. This can best be understood in terms of the dean's responsibility in overseeing the total institutional budget.

In summary, the manner in which money flows into and through the academic medical center has political as well as economic import. In their pursuit of revenues, institutions have begun to operate as interest groups. Through their own efforts and through their professional associations, medical schools have become key participants in the health policy arena.

The Resource Constraint

The decision to finance a new or expanded medical school does not automatically ensure that the essential resources will be available. One of the early constraints on expansion, for example, was a dearth of qualified faculty. This was especially acute prior to the substantial increases in biomedical research funding from the federal government following World War II. This new money served as a magnet for physicians to prepare for careers in teaching and research, facilitating the expansion of faculties in later years.

The supply of teaching patients has been another limitation on expansion. As the undergraduate medical school curriculum has added substantial clinical components, the competition for patients among medical schools in a geographic area and among undergraduate and graduate medical education programs has been heightened.

While there is a broad consensus that medical training ought to be accomplished in the presence of research and patient care, there is little agreement about how much and what kind is necessary to support a given number of medical students. Each institution seeks to cope as best possible, constrained by the resources it is able to marshal.

The Quality Constraint

Intimately related to the issues of cost and resources is the educational quality constraint—the requirement of medical school programs to meet standards established by accrediting agencies. The AMA's Council on Medical Education, which began reviewing medical school standards shortly after the turn of the century, was instrumental in forming the current body, the Liaison Committee on Medical Education, in 1942. The LCME, composed of six AMA Council on Medical Education representatives, six Association of American Medical Colleges Executive Council representatives, two public members, and one federal official, is recognized as an official accrediting agency by the U.S. Office of Education and the National Commission on Accrediting.

From its own perspective, the LCME's activities have influenced medical education expansion efforts in the following manner:

> The accreditation process provides for the medical schools a periodic, external review of assistance to their own efforts in maintaining the quality of their education programs. Outside survey teams are able to focus on the areas of concern which are apparent, recommend other areas requiring increased attention, and indicate areas of strength as well as weakness. In the recent period of major enrollment expansion, the LCME has pointed out to certain schools that the limitations of their resources preclude expanding the enrollment without endangering the quality of the educational program. In yet other cases it has encouraged schools to make more extensive use of their resources to expand their enrollments. During the decade of the sixties particularly, the LCME encouraged and assisted in the development of new medical schools; on the other hand, it has cautioned against the admission of students before an adequate and competent faculty is recruited, or before the curriculum is sufficiently planned and developed and resources gathered for its implementation.[7]

Another mechanism for quality control is state licensure, which historically has had a close kinship with institutional accreditation. The extent to which licensing statutes have incorporated accreditation as a criterion for licensure has led some to conclude that there is now little distinction between the two in practice. Concern has also been voiced about a third element of the interlocking arrangement between accreditation and licensure—eligibility for federal funding. "Accredited or preaccredited status with one of the recognized accrediting bodies," it has been observed, "is established by law as the essential criteria for federal funding, thus giving the accrediting agencies what amounts to a life and death power over the institutions concerned."[8]

The lack of enthusiasm for the expansion of medical education in the 1930s should be viewed in the context of many physicians being underemployed. Julius Richmond has suggested that the memory of privation during the Depression years was vivid in the minds of those later occupying positions of medical leadership, and it may have influenced their position on expanding medical education.[9] While it is always hazardous to attempt to draw direct relationships between the condition of the market for professional services and the level of training capacity—especially in medicine, where so many elements of the competitive market are absent—one should not, however, discount the influence of the market on the leadership.

The dramatic increases in medical school places—on the order of 80 percent over the past decade—has not lessened the suspicion that the AMA has restrained the supply of physicians. Most recently, the Federal Trade Commission's Bureau of Competition challenged the LCME's petition for continued acceptance by the U.S. Office of Education as the official accrediting agency for medical schools. The FTC asserted:

> Accreditation decisions can, when made by representatives of powerful groups with an economic interest in limiting entry into the medical profession, subtly

serve that interest—and therby limit the supply of physicians, deprive some members of the public of access to physician services, and, in general, raise the price of such services and accelerate the already spiraling cost of health care in this country. Nor is the actual existence or nonexistence of biased action the issue; we do not—and need not—assert that AMA or its representatives have in recent years acted improperly with respect to accreditation decisions. The issue is whether there is a conflict, an incentive to act improperly which might be perceived by the public as undermining the fairness of the process.[10]

The LCME managed to retain its recognition for two more years, with the proviso that action be taken to alleviate concerns related primarily to the committee's relationship to the AMA and AAMC.[11]

A more likely explanation is that most professions seek to pursue policies that ensure their dominance, convinced that by such action they are protecting the public. Sometimes they are; often they are protecting themselves. Because of its status, the medical profession has until now been able to enforce its own standards with little restriction. What the future will bring is less clear.

GRADUATE MEDICAL EDUCATION

If all physicians routinely entered practice upon completion of medical school and if physicians were functionally interchangeable, the discussion of the production process could have concluded with the previous analysis. But most physicians undertake additional training to become specialists, and this training affects the character and distribution of the nation's physician supply.

This second stage in the production process transforms medical graduates into specialists. The critical features of the second stage may be outlined briefly as follows:

1. The emergence of a specialty is partly a function of technological developments; thus not all specialties develop at the same time in the same way.
2. The service component of graduate medical education is so substantial that there is on-going conflict and confusion as to whether residents are students or workers.
3. The responsibilities among specialties and between specialists and general practitioners are not clearly demarcated.
4. Graduate medical education has been a major entry point of foreign medical graduates (FMGs) desiring to practice in the United States.

Political conflicts have occurred around the following: attempts to overcome the organizational fragmentation of the governing structure of graduate medical education; conflicts between medical educators and medical practitioners; external pressures to rationalize the distribution of specialties; and attempts to reconcile the dependence on FMGs with an ambivalence over their competence.

Two major voluntary commissions in the 1960s articulated the growing sense that further conciliation and coordination was needed within the medical community. One committee was the AMA-sponsored Citizens Commission on Graduate Education, or the Millis

Commission, after its chairman, John S. Millis, president of Case Western Reserve. A major conclusion of this commission was that a central agency—"responsible to medicine as a whole rather than to particular segments or specialties"—should be created "to secure more unified planning and better articulation of the path" of graduate medical education.[12] Rather forthrightly, the commission report acknowledged that a high order of statesmanship would be required.

> The suggestion that such a central body be established will be interpreted as a threat to the independence of many of the agencies and organizations that now have responsibility for some part of graduate medical education. This interpretation will be correct; the purpose of the proposal is to reduce the independence of a number of existing bodies in order to achieve a more effective and flexible organization.[13]

The second major commission, sponsored by the Association of American Medical Colleges (AAMC), produced what has come to be known as the Coggeshall Report. It has been said that the commission was an influential step in the reorganization of the AAMC, changing its character from "a deans' club, concerned principally with undergraduate medical education, into an association representing the medical schools, specialty societies, and the teaching hospitals."[14] The report advocated "positive and active relationships with key organizations interested in all aspects of education for health and medical sciences."[15] But all this coordination was to take place in the context of the overriding principle expressed by the commission: "Professional physician education should continue in a coordinated sequence under the sponsorship and guidance of university medical schools, through internships and residency programs."[16]

The recommendations of both commissions to provide some mechanism for improvement of graduate medical education eventually became manifest in the form of the Coordinating Council on Medical Education (CCME) and its Liaison Committee on Graduate Medical Education (LCGME), organized in 1972. As the supervisory body over the liaison committees responsible for undergraduate (LCME), graduate (LCGME), and continuing (LCCME) medical education, the CCME must deal with a broad range of cross-cutting policy issues.

The LCGME has responsibility for accrediting programs in graduate medical education based in part on the recommendations made by the residency review committees for each specialty. These review committees are composed of representatives from the AMA's Council on Medical Education, representatives of the particular specialty board, and in some cases representatives of the relevant national specialty society. Membership on the LCGME is shared by five parent organizations (American Board of Medical Specialties, American Hospital Association, American Medical Association, Association of American Medical Colleges, Council of Medical Specialty Societies), as well as having one representative from the public and one from the federal government.[17]

The Coordinating Council on Medical Education has sought to clarify the responsibilities of institutions, organizations, and agencies offering graduate medical education; the supply and distribution of primary-care physicians and foreign medical graduates; the financing of graduate medical education; the impact of national health insurance on medical education; and continuing education for physicians. The nature of these current topics suggests that the two major tensions—conflicts of interest between practitioners and educators over housestaff, and the concomitant struggle among various organizations for control over the accrediting process—are still a part of the general environment within which the key groups operate. Now, however, with the CCME, there exists an organizational framework—although a loose confederation—for confronting differences and agreeing upon mutual objectives.

Some federal government spokesmen are pushing for the CCME to act as the medical profession's major instrument in graduate medical education. In their view, unless the profession regulates itself, the government will be forced to exert direct control over such areas as specialty distribution. While the traditional response of spokesmen for the profession has been that the system is self-regulating and that government interference will only make things worse, there appears to be an active concern among segments of the profession about the future shape of physician supply.

For years, surgeons in particular have served as the whipping boys of the "health-care crisis." On almost everyone's list of the inadequacies of the American health system was the charge that an "oversupply" of surgeons has led to unnecessary surgery. Obviously frustrated by these aspersions, the surgeons decided to sponsor their own study—one representing "the thinking of the surgical community rather than that of some Federal agency or a contractual firm."[18] Thus in 1970, the American College of Surgeons and the American Surgical Association commissioned the Study on Surgical Services for the United States (SOSSUS).[19] A major portion of the $1.5 million study focuses on manpower issues. One of the central conclusions reached was that there is an excess of between 22,000 and 34,000 physicians performing surgery in the United States. The appropriate total, within a range of 50,000 to 60,000, could be reached if only board-certified surgeons were allowed to operate. Clearly, vigorous pursuit of such a goal would create enormous intraprofessional conflict considering the number of non-board-certified physicians who are currently performing surgery.

Another conclusion of the SOSSUS study concerned excessive numbers of surgical residency positions. The authors of the report suggested that the current annual output of surgical residents (2,500 to 3,000) be reduced to 1,600 to 2,000 per year. They acknowledge, however, that without control of hospital privileges to surgeons, monitoring or controlling the number in training becomes meaningless.[20]

There are several basic problems with the SOSSUS study and others like it. Perhaps the major difficulty lies in the state of the art of estimating physician requirements. The problems of projecting manpower needs were illuminated by a study of orthopedic manpower. The authors point out that while a case could be made for 25 percent of the doctor output to enter orthopedics, one can only approximate need without knowing more about the incidence of musculoskeletal conditions in the population and the extent to which other kinds of practitioners treat these problems.[21]

Thus the kinds of assumptions that researchers are forced to make in such a manpower analysis, coupled with the fact that these studies are sponsored by the affected specialty, leave the results open to criticism. The uncertainty is particularly damaging when the findings serve as the basis for administrative action, such as refusing to accredit new programs or eliminating older programs.

The enormity of the taks of intervening in such a complex, interlocking system with the aim of rationalizing the distribution of residencies is one that should be considered not only on the basis of whether we have the knowledge to improve the system, but on an understanding of the political capital required to move the institutions in question. Because graduate medical education policy is so intimately connected with the politics of biomedical research funding and the politics of medical care delivery, a good deal of inertia exists within the system and therefore is likely to frustrate reform. The need for reform does not equate into a successful program of reform: Specialty groups such as surgeons continue to struggle with these difficult problems.

THE RELATIONSHIP BETWEEN UNDERGRADUATE AND GRADUATE MEDICAL EDUCATION

This chapter has presented some of the basic characteristics of two stages of the physician production process: undergraduate and graduate medical education.

As a major though late-blooming force in the medical education policy arena, the Association of American Medical Colleges has been guided by the credo of "the continuum of medical education." This states that the physician can "at no time be considered a finished product, but must now accept continuous education and re-education as a *modus vivendi* inseparable from the application of his skill."[22] Operationally, this has been interpreted to mean that medical schools ought to control all phases of physician education through residency and continuing education.

The president of the Association, Dr. John A. D. Copper, affirmed this principle in an address on the occasion of the one hundredth anniversary of the organization.

> The [AAMC] Assembly adopted the policy that medical school faculties should assume the same responsibility for graduate medical education as they traditionally had for undergraduate medical education. The Association is working on several fronts to implement this policy, which makes eminent sense, given the

increasing integration of undergraduate and graduate medical education and the rapidly developing affiliations between hospitals and medical schools.[23]

The concept of corporate responsibility for graduate medical education has been most vigorously promoted by the AAMC, which adopted a position statement in 1971 and published guidelines in 1973.[24] Academic medical centers are encouraged to develop mechanisms making the entire faculty responsible for graduate medical education and to provide overall administration by administrative teams accountable to an overall governing board that sets broad policy. One of the major effects of such a policy would be to limit the "autonomous discretions" of individual program directors, thus shifting administrative authority to an individual who would assure that "the selection of residents, appointment of faculty, development of curricula, assessment of residency performance, evaluation of the educational process and outcomes, and the commitment of resources for all programs are commensurate with the policies of graduate medical education established by the entire faculty."[25]

The AMA, in its formal approval of the Millis Commission Report, in effect endorsed the idea of corporate responsibility for the medical schools to oversee the entire educational process—undergraduate, graduate, and continuing[26]—and so has the American Hospital Association in its *Statement on Role and Responsibility of Hospitals and Other Health Care Agencies in Health Manpower Education and Training*.[27] A further step was taken when the CCME drafted and approved a statement on corporate responsibility.[28] A preliminary attempt to gauge the progress that academic medical centers are making toward assuming responsibility for graduate medical education was mounted by the AAMC in 1974. A survey of the large majority of U.S. centers revealed that 72 had considered the matter, with 30 of those definitely and 32 probably planning to assume the responsibility.[29]

Some voice skepticism about the ability of medical schools to increase their control over graduate medical education, since the dollars that support such training flow overwhelmingly to the teaching hospitals through reimbursement for patient care. It is a difficult task to overcome the decision-making authority that accompanies such money flows by superimposing an administrative structure—corporate responsibility—that can capture part of these dollars to carry on an improved educational mission.

While public statements have been made in support of the ideal of corporate responsibility from the five major national organizations that constitute the Coordinating Council on Medical Education (CCME), the organizational problems associated with developing policy positions, which must be approved by all the parent bodies, have been considerable. It remains an open question whether either at the institutional level or at the level of national organizations these differences can be resolved.

The foregoing discussion suggests that, while the medical education sector can be conceptualized as a single system, it can also be seen as a loose collection of systems that defies prediction or control. Those who operate within this policy arena have learned to live with multiple contradictions and muddle through accordingly.

The belief that government can influence the physician production process in ways that will ameliorate the deficiencies of the health-care system is the driving force behind most policy initiatives at the state and federal level. In pursuit of this goal, the major task for government has been and will be to discover where it can intervene with greatest positive impact, the most economy of effort, and the largest political gain.

NOTES

1. U.S. Department of Health, Education, and Welfare, Institute of Medicine, *Costs of Education in the Health Professions*, DHEW Publication No. (HRA) 74–32, 1974; Grace M. Carter, et al., *Federal Manpower Legislation and the Academic Health Centers: An Interim Report* (Santa Monica, Ca.: The Rand Corporation, 1974); Rashi Fein and Gerald I. Weber, *Financing Medical Education: An Analysis of Alternative Policies and Mechanisms* (New York: McGraw-Hill, 1971).
2. *Final Report of the Commission on Medical Education*, New York, 1932, p. 283.
3. American Medical Association, "Medical Education in the United States, 1975–1976," *Journal of the American Medical Association*, 27 December 1976, p. 2967.
4. Carter, et al., *Federal Manpower Legislation*, pp. 54–65.
5. Robert G. Petersdorf, "Departments of Medicine—1973," *New England Journal of Medicine*, 29 August 1974, p. 444.
6. Miriam Ostow, "Affiliation Contracts," in *Urban Health Services, The Case of New York*, ed. Eli Ginzberg (New York: Columbia University Press, 1971), pp. 96–118; Robert B. Alford, *Health Care Politics: Ideological and Interest Group Barriers to Reform* (Chicago: University of Chicago Press, 1975).
7. Association of American Medical Colleges, *1975–1976 Annual Report*, Washington, D.C., p. 12.
8. Harold Seidman, "Accreditation of Postsecondary Education: Problems in Organization," in *Study of Accreditation of Selected Health Educational Programs, Staff Working Papers*, Part I, Washington, D.C., 1971, pp. F1–15.
9. Julius B. Richmond, *Currents in American Medicine: A Developmental View of Medical Care and Education* (Cambridge: Harvard University Press, 1969), p. 8.
10. Letter to Edward Aguirre, U.S. Commissioner of Education from Daniel C. Schwartz, Acting Director, Bureau of Competition, Federal Trade Commission, 11 November, 1976, p. 12.
11. Association of American Medical Colleges, *1976–1977 Annual Report*, Washington, D. C., p. 14.
12. Citizens Commission on Graduate Medical Education, *the Graduate Education of Physicians* (Chicago: American Medical Association, 1966), p. 98.
13. Ibid.
14. August G. Swanson, "The Genesis of the Coordinating Council on Medical Education and the Liaison Committee on Graduate Education," *Bulletin of the N.Y. Academy of Medicine* 50 (December 1974): 1219.
15. Lowell T. Coggeshall, *Planning for Medical Progress Through Education* (Evanston: Association of American Medical Colleges, 1965), p. 87.
16. Ibid., p. 39.
17. AMA, "Medical Education 1975–1976," p. 2950.
18. George D. Zuidema, "The Assessment of Issues Facing American Surgery," *Surgery*, (October 1971), p. 496.
19. American College of Surgeons and American Surgical Association, *Surgery in the United States*, 1975.
20. Ibid., p. 85.

21. D. Kay Clawson, et al., *Orthopaedic Manpower Study Phase III*, Committee for the Study of Manpower Requirements in Orthopaedic Surgery, 1974, pp. 26–27.

22. Coggeshall, *Planning for Medical Progress*, pp. 39–40.

23. John A. D. Cooper, "The Association of American Medical Colleges: Looking Ahead from the First Hundred Years," *Journal of Medical Education* 52 (January 1977): 15.

24. Committee on Graduate Medical Education, "Guidelines."

25. Ibid., p. 786.

26. Citizens Commission, *Graduate Education of Physicians*, pp. 60–61.

27. "Graduate Medical Education: Moving Toward a New Status Quo," *Hospitals*, 16 August 1974, p. 42.

28. Tom E. Nesbitt, "The Coordinating Council on Medical Education: A Progress Report in the Pursuit of Acceptance of Responsibility," *Journal of the Tennessee Medical Association* 68 (March 1975): 195.

29. August Swanson and Mary H. Littlemeyer, "Academic Medical Centers and Graduate Medical Education," *Journal of Medical Education* 50 (April 1975): 409–11.

3

The Federal Role: Congress

Having examined the structure of the medical education sector, we now turn to explore the role of the federal government: Specifically, what led to political intervention in responding to the physician shortage and what was the nature of the response. Further, how did Congress view the states' continuing role in the expansion of medical education?

THE FEDERAL GOVERNMENT AND THE MEDICAL EDUCATION SECTOR

The Health Professions Educational Assistance Act of 1963 united the medical education sector and the federal government in a marriage of convenience in which each party saw the potential fulfillment of its own ends. The principal goal of the medical education sector was to gain greater financial stability. The federal government was determined to increase the output of physicians on the presumption that this was a necessary step in the improvement of the health-care-delivery system. Although these two objectives were in many ways complementary, the divergence of purposes was sufficiently great to produce continuing frustrations and conflict.

The interface between the medical education sector and health care and health research was not taken into account in designing how federal funds would be used to achieve the desired expansion. More physicians would ultimately solve improved coverage for the underserved. When this was realized, the exploration of ways in which the production process might address the important problem of access moved to center stage. In this connection, the nation's medical schools were perceived as having a claim on federal tax dollars to help assure the continued and expanded output of physicians. However, this was not valid as a claim for full funding, but rather for up-front dollars.

The medical education community, skeptical at first of a physician shortage, became attracted to the view that the medical system could be reformed through the education process. Medical education was to become more humane, more innovative, and involved in the delivery of services. It was to attack problems by reaching out into the community. Lately this enthusiasm has been somewhat dampened. Although medical educators will not return to the insulation of an earlier period, they have become more cautious about providing help because of the fear that they will be held accountable for failing to bring about changes beyond the limits of their abilities.

The overlapping and divergence of medical schools and federal imperatives deserve further elaboration, particularly as they relate to the financial stabilization of medical schools and legislative efforts to employ federal dollars to expand the physician production process.

Prelude to Congressional Action

The first program of direct federal support for medical education in 1963 reflects calculations of what was politically possible in light of the failures of the past attempts of federal intervention. The passage of the Health Professions Education Assistance Act of 1963 was preceded by efforts in the early 1950s, when such a program appeared likely to pass. Stephen Strickland recounts the first major congressional attempt to deal with these problems. In September 1949, the Senate passed a five-year emergency program of grants and scholarships to health professional schools. The measure, however, died in the Rules Committee. By the time Congress was ready to meet again, the AMA's original "tentative support" had been transformed into "outright opposition" on the advice of their advertising representatives Whitaker and Baxter, who saw hidden threats looming behind federal aid to medical education. According to Strickland, the AMA succeeded in killing the 1950–51 proposals by enlisting the services of Senator Everett Dirksen, key physicians who were encouraged to influence their congressmen, and, perhaps most importantly, Senator Robert Taft, who in the previous Congress had been one of the major Republican supporters of the original bill. The final blow to passage was dissension among the medical school deans over a provision that would have largely benefited the less prestigious schools by emphasizing incentive money for expanded enrollment rather than financial need (some of the more renowned medical colleges were in particularly difficult financial straits).[1]

Elton Rayack characterizes the AMA stance over the period of 1951-57 as one of "strategic retreat in the face of continued pressure." The organization cautiously supported federal assistance for construction but denied the existence of a physician shortage. The AMA acknowledged that distribution might be a problem but behind that the addition of 361 [sic] doctors to the supply would solve it. The "overwhelming sense of urgency" created by the Bayne-Jones Report (1958), the Bane Report (1959), and the Jones Report in 1960 led to "a gradual but full retreat" on the part of the AMA with respect to its position on the doctor shortage.[2]

By 1963, the AMA position had become one of support for construction and public neutrality—tempered with last-minute, behind-the-scenes opposition—on the question of student loans. One observer at the time noted that the AMA's opposition to the loan program seemed "relatively perfunctory as compared to its campaign against medical care for the aged."[3] Nonetheless, once it was clear that the AMA had accepted the principle of some kind of program of federal aid for medical education, congressional leaders could proceed with building a consensus for a specific piece of legislation.

The brittleness of that consensus is revealed by Senator Listor Hill's comment during the debate in his defense of the committee's decision to oppose amendments on the floor: "The problem is to pass this basic legislation now . . . then be in a position to propose any changes or any amendments that we see fit to propose."[4]

The bargaining inherent in the process of building majorities in Congress militates against a comprehensive attack on social problems. The long history of conflict in this arena dictated that modest rather than revolutionary attempts to deal with the problems would have to suffice. In the case of the 1963 legislation, issues of geographic and specialty distribution, increasing reliance upon foreign medical graduates, and operational support for medical schools were relegated to the background, while two other questions were being resolved—namely, whether there was a *need* for a massive new infusion of public monies and whether it was *proper* for the federal government to provide such support. Thus the consensus eventually achieved in Congress was based on a belief that the physician shortage was dangerous to a point where federal assistance was required.

Construction of medical school facilities and student loans proved to be an acceptable expression of congressional consensus—a consensus that would have been virtually impossible to create had there been an attempt, as in later years, to deal more directly with altering the character of the supply of physicians. As Senator Hill predicted, once the legislation was on the statute books, a continuing process of modification would be set in motion, reflecting, if not always deeper understanding of the problems, at least greater willingness to expand the federal role to promote solutions to whatever problems seemed most pressing.

Througout the 1960s and into the 1970s, the overriding—but not exclusive—federal concern was with increasing the supply of physicians. The conception of what was needed to encourage the desired increases broadened from money for "bricks and mortar" to various kinds of institutional support and incentive grants. Attitudes toward student assistance also changed. And, moreover, a greater federal role was beginning to be discussed as a means of improving health care in underserved areas, encouraging the training of primary-care practitioners, and altering medical school curricula to prepare students for changing patterns of health-care delivery.

THE FINANCIAL STABILITY OF MEDICAL SCHOOLS

One of the early danger signals pointing to the need for federal assistance was the growing awareness of the deepening financial crisis facing medical education.

As early as 1948, President Truman's Federal Security Administrator, Oscar Ewing, noted in a report based on the proceedings of the National Health Assembly that medical colleges would have difficulty in achieving the double task of expanding enrollments and improving the quality of instruction: "At the present time, many medical and health educational institutions are so crippled by lack of funds that they can do neither. Under the pressure of rising enrollments, many need financial assistance even to maintain present standards."[5]

Reports and pronouncements by various interest groups centered on the dire financial outlook. Appeals to the business community by voluntary National Fund for Medical Education, Inc., forcefully conveyed the message that medical schools were "staggering under a growing financial burden" and that their deficits were imperiling the nation's health.[6] The higher-education community expressed its alarm at the disproportionate share of funds medical schools were drawing from overall university budgets. The Association of American Universities reported in 1951 from its study of medical school financing: "A sampling of 18 private universities and 18 public universities points up the fact that medical education constitutes the most pressing single financial problem of those institutions of higher learning which have a medical school."[7]

The President's Commission on the Health Needs of the Nation lent further credence to these disquieting statistics by highlighting the financial problems of medical schools in their report, *building America's Health.* The report noted that practically no medical school had been able to meet its budget out of current income.[8]

A major effort was launched by Rep. Oren Harris, Chairman of the Interstate and Foreign Commerce Committee, in 1957, to "gather all possible information bearing on the subject of federal aid to medical education."[9] The committee staff discovered what others previously—and since—have discovered in the pursuit of information on the financing of medical education.

1. Medical school operating expenses were increasing at an enormous rate.

2. Tuition income contributes a smaller and smaller portion of total operating expenses: 22.5 percent in 1950–1 and 18.2 percent in 1956–7.

3. There is no uniform pattern with regard to the cost of teaching as reported by medical schools ($1,000 to $15,000 per student in 1959).

4. It is difficult to measure accurately the cost of teaching medical students, because
   (a) medical schools receive supplies, services and funds from their parent universities;
   (b) the interrelated function of research and patient care are integral parts of the medical education program;
   (c) medical schools are also involved in graduate and continuing education programs.[10]

In the early Senate and House Reports of 1962 and 1963, the concept of medical schools as a "national resource" was acknowledged. However, in view of the AMA's public rationalization of its acceptance of federal aid as a one-time expenditure, the idea of the federal government providing continuing institutional support was not openly discussed. Instead, the argument in support of federal aid was framed in the following manner: "Without such assistance at this time we seriously jeopardize our great investment in medical research and health facilities."[11] The point to be made is that this new form of federal aid did not differ from the well-established Hill-Burton and NIH support programs; but an adequate supply of manpower was needed to staff hospitals and utilize research findings.

The AAMC, while not wishing to jeopardize the first legislative intervention by pushing for outright institutional support, was poised to move in that direction. The association had in 1961 adopted the following position:

> But this program alone will not provide enough physicians to meet the needs of the Nation. A strong system of medical education requires adequate financial support that is continuing and stable. Universities with budgets already under great stress will be unable to maintain, improve, or expand their existing medical programs or to establish new medical schools or new educational programs unless sources of additional operating funds are found.[12]

The AMA was not attempting to hide the financial plight of medical schools. A 1962 report by its Council on Medical Education called attention to the fact that many schools needed increased funds for construction and operating costs, even to maintain current enrollment levels. Of special concern were so-called have-not schools, since their financial problems were, as the CME concluded, "so serious that their educational programs are being compromised." However, one of the messages of the report was a warning against "overdependence of a medical school on any one source of funds. . . . When that source is the federal government with all its potential for external control, the concern is even greater."[13]

The Health Professions Educational Assistance Act of 1963, devoid of funds for operational support, could be viewed mainly as the promise of better things to come—the thin edge of the wedge. The provisions for construction money and student aid in some cases, however, could help avert short-run financial crises. For those medical schools in dire need of renovations of inefficient facilities, the construction funding was important not only for what it could achieve directly but also as a line to raising additional monies from other sources. Choosing to ignore the AMA's warnings about the danger of federal control, the House Committee, however, quoted from the AMA's report to demonstrate the need for basic improvement grants to strengthen curriculum and faculty in the have-not schools.[14]

Those arguing against these grants on the floor of the House contended that a serious precedent was being set for all of higher education by providing direct operating support to medical schools. The proponents countered by citing the support of land-grant colleges; medical schools were also serving clear and pressing national needs. For one thing, medical graduates were highly mobile and settled in all parts of the country. For another, about 12 percent of the nation's physicians were on full-time duty in the Department of Defense, the Public Health Service, and the Veterans Administration.[15]

The nub of the arguments in favor of improvement grants rested on the precarious position of the ten to twelve schools supposedly on the brink of financial disaster. Committee Chairman Oren Harris argued:

> How can we say we are going to establish a program, as we are providing in this bill, to increase the number of medical institutions by at least 10 new schools and then permit a dozen old established medical schools to go by the way. It just is not practicable.[16]

Remembering the dissension among the medical school ranks in the 1950s, which prevented the passage of aid to medical education at that time, the 1965 proposals were carefully constructed. The "fortunate medical schools" could use the money to pioneer in developing experimental programs, while the others could use the money to keep their heads above water.

Deliberation of the next round of health manpower legislation in 1968 followed in the wake of a prestigious National Advisory Commission on Health Manpower, established by President Lyndon Johnson in 1966. Among its many recommendations, the commission urged consideration of a program of direct federal support for the educational function of medical schools. Institutional rather than categorical support would allow educational officers some flexibility in modernizing curricula and expanding enrollment.[17]

The 1968 law saw Congress moving further in this direction: Basic improvement grants were renamed "institutional grants," and each school with an approved application received a minimum of $25,000 per year, plus additional funds to be distributed on a formula basis, rewarding those schools with the greatest enrollment increases. Congressional discomfort over have-not schools was still high, and the new, improved special-improvement grants were designed to save these floundering institutions. Thus changes were made in the provisions of the law relating to special improvement grants: (1) there would no longer be a statutory ceiling on these grants; (2) the Secretary of HEW would be required to give consideration to the relative need of the schools; and (3) if circumstances warranted, schools unable to raise 50 percent matching funds for construction could be eligible for up to 66 and two-thirds percent from the federal government.

In 1971, during the Health Professions Education Assistance Act hearings, Congress heard a replay of the familiar plaint of medical schools on the brink of financial chaos. Dr. William Analyan, representing the AAMC, announced that "the financial crisis that long has been predicted has arrived at last—and with a vengeance." The magnitude of that crisis was described as follows:

> During fiscal 1970, 61 of the 102 medical schools sought special grants from NIH to offset financial distress. In thirty-two of these instances, the financial problems were so serious that the continued operation or accreditation of the schools was threatened. Johns Hopkins University School of Medicine in Baltimore is a case in point. It is one of the oldest, most prestigious, and apparently most wealthy medical schools in the country. Yet in past weeks, the State of Maryland has had to extend $800,000 of emergency financial aid, just to enable Hopkins to survive.[18]

Whereas for years Congress had heard that eight to ten medical schools were moribund, the critical list had risen to thirty-two by 1971. To make matters worse, Johns Hopkins—that school upon which the Flexnerian ideal was based—appeared to be in serious trouble.

Part of the solution to this problem of financial instability was seen in greater direct federal funding of instructional costs. The recommendations of the Carnegie Commission on Higher Education came at a strategic moment in the legislative process and quickly gained the support of HEW, OMB, and interest groups like the AAMC. Among the well-publicized recommendations—the call for a 52-percent increase in medical school entrants achieved the most attention—was the suggestion that the federal government should adopt a cost-of-instruction supplement to institutions.[19] The concept of supplements eventually developed into capitation grants. The major controversy during the legislative process of operationalizing this type of support was over how large these grants should be and whether the federal government should undertake a first-dollar or a last-dollar approach to funding. In the end, the first-dollar approach prevailed. Grace Carter and her colleagues at the Rand Corporation have provided a perspective on this first-dollar/last-dollar issue:

> . . . [financial distress] grants placed the federal government in the position of providing residual financing ("last dollar" financing). . . . The choice was one between a targeted program in which the schools had to justify their needs to the federal government, and a formula grant program in which each school would be given a basic grant to spend as it pleased.[20]

It was recognized that capitation alone would not solve the financial problems of many schools. Secretary of HEW, Elliot Richardson, explained to Congress in his testimony why the Administration believed a separate authority for financial distress grants was needed:

> Mr. Chairman, financial distress is a commonly used term today, but is less commonly understood. Financial distress may, or may not be related to the educational process. . . . Although the Administration's capitation grant program will contribute significantly to the alleviation of financial distress in schools of medicine, osteopathy, and dentistry, a number of these schools may need temporary financial assistance before their fiscal problems can be solved.[21]

The Secretary of HEW was charged with the responsibility of determining the need for financial assistance to medical schools and reporting his findings to Congress. In attempting these cost studies, HEW encountered the problem of allocating costs among teaching, research, and patient care. The need for comparable cost data, as well as the need for consistent accounting techniques, was highlighted. To that end, the 1971 law required schools to agree to three stipulations in order to receive financial distress grants: (1) disclose any financial information deemed necessary by the Secretary of HEW: (2) conduct comprehensive analysis studies; and (3) carry out appropriate financial and operational reforms. Schools preferred to make do with the new capitation and other project grants. Whereas 200 applications for distress grants from medical schools were funded between 1968 and 1971, only 10 grantees took advantage of the program between FY 1972 and FY 1974.[22]

The lengthy dispute in the 92d Congress (1971) over how much capitation medical schools should receive led to the inclusion of Section 205 in the law, which instructed the Secretary of HEW to arrange for a study to determine the national annual-per-student educational cost of health profession schools. The Institute of Medicine (IOM) of the National Academy of Sciences was charged with the responsibility for conducting the study.

Like earlier groups, the IOM uncovered a wide range in education expenditures. The annual student cost of instruction for medical schools was found to vary between $5,150 and $14,150, with an average of $9,700. The study concluded that capitation payments *authorized* under the 1971 Act amounted to between 25 and 40 percent of the average *net* education expenditures—about the amount required to stabilize the financial condition of the schools. However, appropriation levels for the capitation grants fluctuated each year and fell below authorized amounts.[23]

The IOM endorsed the policy of a capitation grant program as "an appropriate Federal undertaking to provide a stable source of support for health professional schools." Several reasons were advanced:

1. The relationship between the health-care delivery system and the performance of the schools in providing for national health manpower needs.
2. The need to prevent a condition of financial distress among the schools.
3. The value of medical schools as a national resource considering the geographic distribution of schools in relation to population and the mobility of health professionals.
4. The possible negative effects of increased pressure on states to assume a

large burden for private medical school financing and consequently greater control over institutional policies.

5. The need for institutions to have a predictable and stable source of income so they can plan and manage their programs.[24]

The study group also concluded that capitation was probably not an effective tool for achieving such objectives as improved geographic and specialty distribution. Its reasoning served to fortify the view of medical schools as a "national resource" deserving of general federal support irrespective of other national goals that the schools may be asked to address.

Despite these recommendations, the mood of the Administration and of many of those in Congress was shifting away from unconditional institutional support. For example, after acknowledging the progress made under HPEA, Assistant Secretary Charles Edwards expressed this viewpoint in 1974 congressional hearings:

> However, the Federal health manpower programs have utilized and generated a demand for considerable fiscal resources and have tended to create a serious dependence on the Federal Government. The ready availability of Federal funds, including Medicare and Medicaid reimbursement, has produced limited cost consciousness in health professional schools, and, accordingly, we have seen the cost of such education rise substantially.[25]

The Assistant Secretary went on to speak of the dangers of an oversupply of physicians and the need to target federal support on improved distribution and more efficient use of paramedical personnel.

At about this time, Senator Edward Kennedy, as chairman of the Health Subcommittee, began to push for medical school accountability. The following excerpt from the Senate report on the unsuccessful 1974 proposals illustrates this:

> This committee believes that the public at large is *not* receiving full value. . . . However, this committee wishes to explicitly point out that, if it cannot in good conscience have confidence in programs intended to effectively overcome these problems, that it will be forced to conclude that these funds can be more wisely expended for other purposes.[26]

Although the authorization for the Comprehensive Health Manpower Act of 1971 had expired in 1974, Congress was unable to agree on new legislation. In the process of existing on continuing resolutions, the amount each school received was continually eroded by inflation, by reduced appropriations, and by the fact that newer schools became eligible to compete for a shrinking pot of money. The level of formula grants, for example, declined from $106 million in FY 1974 to $86 million in FY 1975.[27]

AAMC president John A. D. Cooper painted a bleak picture of the financial future of medical schools when he presented his report at the 1974 assembly in Chicago. He listed among the problems facing the medical education sector: concentrating federal research funds into contract research centers, confusing and conflicting regulations of the health-care industry, skyrocketing inflation, and complex requirements attached to capitation grants, "which threatened to bankrupt the institutions attempting to carry them out." The ill effects of these forces on the quality of education programs could be measured by the decrease in the average term of accreditation. "The rapid increase in enrollments, the inadequacy of financial resources, the turnover in deans and department chairman, and the dilution of the faculty pool by new schools," said Cooper, "are all contributing factors."[28] The AAMC, in its own proposal on capitation, suggested an annual grant of $3,250 per student, about half of which would be unrestricted, while the remainder would require certain target efforts on the part of the medical school.[29]

The 1974 bills died in conference at the close of the 93d Congress, but by July 1975 the House managed to approve a bill similar to the previous year's proposal. Congressman Paul Rogers, chairman of the substantive House subcommittee and viewed as less threatening to the AAMC's position than either the Administration or Senator Kennedy, nonetheless often expressed the opinion that medical schools should make good on their claim of being a national resource by agreeing to address shortages and distributional problems. Unlike most of the other engaged parties, Rogers still argued, in 1975, that enrollments needed to be increased even further to meet future requirements of a national health insurance program as well as to reduce reliance on FMGs.[30]

Although the Administration talked for some time about weaning the medical schools away from capitation support, this form of assistance had the virtue of providing a vehicle for attaching strings to proposals of interest to involved congressmen. The strings were usually designed to address geographic and specialty maldistribution; i.e., remote site training, regulatory mechanisms for controlling residency slots, requirements for schools to set aside portions of their first-year classes for those willing to practice in shortage areas. The bone of contention between Congress and medical education leaders was over how much it would cost schools to institute these innovations. Congress would not pay directly but would expect the schools to support themselves on their capitation allowance. Questions of interfering with the independence of schools and the government's need for accountability in the use of the taxpayers' money also added spice to the policy debate.

Politically this translated into a flurry of activity, which was described by *Science*:

> It was late in July [1976] before the Senate finally managed to pass a manpower bill, and then it took several weeks for a House-Senate conference. During this time, medical school administrators were going crazy with fear that no bill would be passed before Congress adjourned for the elections and the capitation funds on which they have come to rely might not be forthcoming. Deans, and even university presidents, by the dozens came to town to lobby for or against this or that provision in somebody's bill.[31]

In the end, capitation levels were set at $2,000 in FY 1978, increasing to $2,100 by FY 1980. To qualify, schools would be required to maintain at least first-year enrollment levels, work toward filling 50 percent of their first-year affiliated residency positions in primary care, and reserve places for qualified U.S. students who had completed two years at a foreign medical school. While the worst fears of the medical education community were not incorporated into the legislation, this last measure was seen as a flagrant violation of the rights of institutions to select their own students.

As an alternative to institutional support, there has been increased interest in shifting the locus of accountability from medical schools to medical students. By providing substantial loan and scholarship support while at the same time reducing capitation funds, schools will be forced to raise tuition, obliging students to accept federal financial support tied to service paybacks. Institutional support would be limited then to project grants to deal with special problems, such as increasing primary-care physicians.

Despite more than two decades of serious debate over how involved the federal government should be in the finances of medical schools, no stable relationship has emerged. When the deans talk about their medical schools as a national resource, it sounds as though they were describing a national forest that should be allowed to flourish in its pristine beauty under the protection of the federal government. On the other hand, Congress has sometimes appeared to view the medical schools as though their output were comparable to that of the aerospace industry. The medical school representatives are sometimes chastised as though they were Lockheed executives who have just delivered a fleet of outmoded bombers at huge cost overruns.

The exigencies of the political process, however, have forced compromises. The medical education interests have begun to appreciate the budgetary and accountability considerations and to understand—although not fully—the aversion of Congress to subsidize institutions that produce the highest-paid professionals. It is easier to sell Congress programs designed to solve widely perceived problems—whether it be shortages or maldistribution—than programs designed to support institutions.

Congress was interested, in one respect at least, in the financial well-being of medical schools primarily as it related to their productive capacity and concern over the quality of their product. One powerful argument was that it did not make sense to start new medical schools while permitting old ones to succumb.

For individual congressmen, however, there was a good deal of sympathy for the stringent financial conditions of the schools. Just as the average citizen may view the AMA with considerable suspicion but invest a great deal of trust in his own family doctor, the local medical school may be a source of considerable pride and concern for the legislator, even though he may concurrently hold critical views about the performance of the medical education sector as a whole. Furthermore, in many cases, medical schools and their parent universities may wield considerable influence among a legislator's constituency.

GEOGRAPHIC MALDISTRIBUTION

From the outset, Congress recognized that the physician supply was unevenly distributed geographically. Initially, this was expressed mainly as a problem of rural constituencies. As a senator from North Dakota observed in the 1963 *Congressional Record*: "I have had a constant problem, year after year, in trying to help small communities to try to find doctors. My hometown, having a population of about 1,000, has had to depend, for the most part, on doctors from Canada."[32] Another congressman describes his 14-year effort at securing a physician for his county: "We bought him a cattle ranch. We already had plenty of patients for him. We got him out of the Air Force. He stayed just long enough to see if he was clear of the Air Force. Then he left our people high and dry."[33]

While it became popular in the mid-1970s to berate earlier Congresses for their naivete concerning the relationship of expanding total supply to physician migration patterns, at least one congressman, as early as 1963, was aware of the need to deal more directly with the problem:

> There is very little evidence that there is a shortage of either dentists or doctors in the cities. Unless we can provide some method of getting doctors and dentists into the areas where there is a shortage—and those are the rural areas—then I must confess that there is not much evidence in the hearings which would support the stated purposes of the entire bill.[34]

The House report accompanying its 1963 bill acknowledged that physician shortages were particularly acute in small communities and rural areas of the nation. An HEW study had revealed that in 1960, one-third of the counties in the United States had more than 2,000 people per physician; whereas one physician for 1,000 persons was considered necessary for comprehensive medical care.[35]

As the committee saw it, one measure to help solve this problem was the inclusion of a forgiveness feature in its loan program. If a student practiced in a shortage area designated by the state health authority, 50 percent of the unpaid principal and interest on the loan would be canceled at a rate of 10 percent a year. The committee also thought that the establishment of new medical schools in states currently without them would also help alleviate the problem, since students would be more likely to remain in or be attracted to states where there was a medical school with a teaching hospital.[36]

It was not until 1965 that a majority of the House was prepared to pass a loan-forgiveness measure. Opposition was partly because of jurisdictional disputes between the Commerce Committee and the Education and Labor Committee, the latter being afraid that this might be a poor precedent. Others arguing against the bill expressed the view that big government could not buy willingness to practice or serve, that it was more logical to travel 50 miles to expert care on good roads than 5 miles to less qualified care, and that many states with forgiveness loans up to 60 percent had failed to attract doctors in outlying areas.[37]

The proponents—many with rural constituencies—felt that the measure was, as Congressman Kenneth Roberts of Alabama described it, "a very moderate way of saying to the people who live in rural communities that we are going to try to get some doctors to get out and serve your needs."

For the next several years, Congress did not deal specifically with the question of distribution. However, in the meanwhile, the President's National Advisory Commission on Health Manpower sought to analyze the problem from a broader perspective:

> Many health problems of the disadvantaged are not susceptible of solution by dollars alone or by traditional health programs. Because the demand for health services will continue to exceed supply, simply increasing aggregate resources will not entice health personnel away from the more affluent areas in which they and their families prefer to live and work.[38]

The commission recommended new, experimental programs to deal with the special problems of the disadvantaged. In essence, it pointed out that successful innovation required the cooperation of the private sector, a willingness to risk failure, and the capability to extract worthwhile elements from experiments and to try again.

The issue of geographic maldistribution re-emerged in the 1971 legislation. Taking their cue indirectly from the President's Advisory Commission and more directly from the Carnegie Report, the legislators began to think more in terms of projects and experiments.

The House committee declared in its report that it was "particularly concerned to find ways and means of encouraging and stimulating changes in distribution, as well as increasing numbers, of trained health professions personnel."[39] And the Senate said: "It is the intention of this Committee to assure, to the extent possible, that no county in any of the United States is without the services of a practicing, resident physician."[40]

Several approaches were included in the law (P.L. 92-157) in an attempt to achieve these goals:

> Forgiveness loans were to be cancelled at the higher rate of 30 percent for each of the first two years of service and 25 percent for the third year.
>
> Scholarship grants of up to $5,000 per academic year to those students practicing in shortage areas or in areas primarily serving migratory, agricultural workers.
>
> Medical education initiative awards to be used for the purpose of identifying and enrolling persons who would practice in rural areas.
>
> Special project grants for improving geographic distribution.
>
> Assignment of Public Health Service doctors to counties without physicians.
>
> National Health Manpower Shortage Clearinghouse to help match professionals and communities with manpower needs.

Two key programs aimed at distributing health professionals more evenly developed from Congress in 1970 and 1971: the National Health Service Corps and the Area Health Education Center program.

A detailed, personalized account of the passage of the National Health Service Corps (NHSC) bill has been offered by Eric Redman in his *Dance of Legislation*. Envisioned as an "experiment rather than a panacea," the original conception of the bill was described by Redman:

> The NHSC would therefore be something of a "marriage bureau" for doctors and needy areas: volunteers would be paid by government during a trial period in the Corps, and then they and the community could decide whether to make the arrangement permanent, either through the establishment of a standard private practice or through the creation of a "health care delivery team" composed of socially motivated health professionals.[41]

The idea for a doctor corps was not new: Such a proposal had been recommended by the President's Commission on Rural Poverty in 1967 and as long ago as the 1930s by Senator Huey Long.[42]

The idea for the Area Health Education Center (AHEC) concept has been attributed to the Carnegie Commission Report of 1970, which described the AHECs:

> The Commission recommends the development of area health education centers in areas of some distance from university health science centers which do not have sufficiently large populations to support university health science centers of their own, and in a few metropolitan areas needing additional training facilities but not full health science centers.[43]

Congress viewed the Health Manpower Education Initiative Awards, of which AHEC was a part, as a way "to target support for health manpower training activities in areas of greatest need and across disciplinary lines." AHECs were to provide "opportunities for the exposure of medical students, interns, residents, and other health professionals to delivery of health care in the community—a major step toward directing training efforts toward places where the real problems are."[44] This view was consistent with that of the Administration (which took the initiative in backing the AHEC concept). The Administration conceived of AHECs and HMOs as part of a long-range strategy toward directing health manpower resources to areas of critical shortage.[45]

While the targeted efforts of the 1971 Act have continued to be funded, consideration of new legislation beginning in 1974 evidenced a restless state among congressional leaders as to whether more direct measures were needed to deal with the distribution problem. The question was whether to focus directly on the students via strong monetary inducements through the National Health Service Corps or, alternatively, to exert leverage on the schools. The latter route was favored by Senator Kennedy, who sought to place the burden on the schools for guaranteeing that a portion of their students would accept National Health Service Corps scholarships. In the end, the focus was mostly on the student; however, the compromise within Congress involved a complicated "trigger" device whereby funding for the scholarship program would be guaranteed (in a fashion) through a mechanism of tying the fate of scholarship appropriations to capitation appropriations.

IMPROVED SPECIALTY DISTRIBUTION

Shortly before Congress began debating the HPEA Act of 1963, an article appeared in *U.S. News and World Report.* The often-quoted article, entitled "Shortage of Doctors—What's Causing It," neatly sums up the thinking of the time:

> The shortage of family doctors seems to be getting worse. Two counties out of three need more physicians. Many hospitals stay open only with the aid of foreign medical trainees. What's wrong? Authorities' view: Research is luring too many medical men and teaching staffs from the goal of everyday medical practice.[46]

Legislators today would probably agree with all but the last sentence—the answer to "What's wrong?" Many would argue that it is not necessarily research that is luring doctors away from everyday practice, but the desire to practice lucrative, esoteric medicine and surgery.

The oversupply of specialty practitioners was not a great worry in the 1950s and early 1960s. Any attention paid to specialty practice mainly concentrated on the subject of a shortage of psychiatrists and pediatricians. For example, the National Health Assembly (1948) had called for an increase in the number of psychiatrists from 4,500 to 15,000 and of pediatricians from 3,500 to 10,500.[47]

While it was recognized in the immediate post-World War II era that specialists were proliferating, it was not considered bad (except by the accrediting bodies concerned with maintaining high-quality programs). President Truman's Commission on the Health Needs of the Nation declared that the specialist must be regarded "as one of the most important health resources in the Nation."[48] In general, the commission viewed increasing specialization as a natural response to the more scientific and complex character of medicine. On the other hand, while recognizing the continuing positive role of the general practitioner, the commission clearly left an impression of uncertainty about his capabilities:

> Since there are no direct and few indirect controls over the scope of work these physicians undertake, it is to be expected that a significant number will attempt work beyond their capacity thus exposing a section of the population to unnecessary and undesirable medical hazards.[49]

During the early 1960s, there was a great deal of agitation within the profession (especially by the American Academy of General Practice [AAGP]) to elevate the status of general practitioners. This agitation led to a number of commission reports, including the AMA's "Meeting the Challenge of Family Practice," and eventually to the establishment in 1969 of a certifying board for family practice. Concurrently, the notion that the specialization trend might have some undesirable consequences was spreading. The authors of the President's Advisory Committee on Health Manpower observed: "Specialization has decreased the number of physicians available to provide care for the entire family and has resulted in a reduction in the number of persons seen per physician."[50]

In 1970, the AAGP succeeded in garnering congressional support for a bill to provide grants for the establishment of separate and distinct departments of family medicine in medical schools. The bill passed both houses of Congress, but not without the opposition of HEW and the AAMC, both of whom opposed the categorical nature of the bill. The AAGP pointed out the irony of such objections on the part of NIH and AAMC, "who have prospered magnificently by dispersing and receiving substantial funds for categorical research." The "bureaucrats and their allies in the medical research/administrative teaching complex" (in the AAGP vernacular) won out, for President Nixon succeeded in a controversial "pocket veto" to scuttle the program.[51]

The setback was only temporary, however, for in the Comprehensive Health Manpower Training Act of 1971 a family medicine grant program was established. These grants were to be awarded to teaching hospitals for the development, expansion, or improvement of or participation in family-practice residency training programs.

While the move to enhance the status of the general practitioner was taking hold, a concurrent trend of critically assessing the role of specialty medicine in the health-care system was developing. In particular, Senator Kennedy has repeatedly emphasized the theme of specialty imbalances, which would lead to serious consequences for the health-care consumer. The basis for much of this criticism has been the work of such researchers as John P. Bunker and Charles E. Lewis, both of whom have demonstrated a relationship between the number of surgeons and the number of surgical operations performed.[52] Kennedy has been supported in this line of attack by HEW officials.

As in the case of geographic maldistribution, the problem of specialty distribution does not lend itself to easy solutions. The complexity of graduate medical education has been discussed in Chapter 2. Whether one chooses to rely on incentives, regulation, or a combination of both, the inevitable questions of "How much will it cost?" and "Who will do it?" present complex political dilemmas.

These questions were considered during the congressional debate on the Health Professions Educational Assistance Act of 1976. The final compromise emerged as a curious amalgam of incentives and regulation—incentives that for practical purposes cannot be refused. While Senator Kennedy wanted a national council to establish goals for the number of first-year residents entering each medical specialty, the aim being to achieve a 50 percent ratio between primary-care physicians and specialists, Congressman Rogers preferred a more indirect, voluntary approach. As finally enacted, the law mandates that the nation's medical schools, as a group, reach the 50-percent level for first-year affiliated residencies by 1980. If the schools as a group do not reach the goal, they will then be responsible on an individual basis for meeting the quota at the risk of losing their capitation.

In addition to these provisions, emphasis was also placed on encouraging the develoment of family medicine through project grants and student aid.

SUBSIDIARY GOALS

Aside from the major goals of producing greater numbers of primary-care physicians for underserved areas, related objectives can be identified in the legislative history. One important area—beyond the scope of this study, but deserving mention—is the parallel encouragement by Congress of expanding other health professional groups. Most notable is the support for advanced training for nurses and the development of training programs for physician assistants. Congress looked to these ancillary health manpower personnel to increase the productivity or substitute for more physicians in shortage areas. While there is evidence that the discriminating use of such personnel saves physician time and reduces cost, it has been suggested that "too little is known about the relative costs and benefits of large-scale replication of the many diverse training programs."[53]

Another goal of Congress has been to use the leverage of federal support to improve the opportunity of certain groups to enter the medical profession. Much of what has been accomplished in the way of increasing the proportion of minority students and women, however, has been through legal and administrative actions embedded in the Equal Employment Opportunity program. The financial aid offered through health manpower legislation has served to support these trends.

Because of the current pressure to enter medical school, it seems incredible that in 1963 there was widespread concern that medical schools were having difficulty filling their classes with well-qualified students. Yet this was what Congress heard in testimony from the Secretary of HEW Anthony Celebreze:

> What I am saying now is that because of lack of expansion facilities, we cannot increase the number of medical students as we want to, and second, we do not even have the choice that we would like to have as to quality, because so many students who are very capable are going into other professions.[54]

In addition to the expected benefit of attracting high-quality students, there was interest in opening up medical schools to lower-income groups. President Kennedy, referring to the difficulty schools were having in securing qualified applicants who could afford the heavy financial burden of medical education, noted that while college enrollments had been rising, the number of applicants to medical schools had been dropping. "It is not surprising," said the President, "that 40 percent of all medical students now come from the 12 percent of the families with incomes of $10,000 or more a year."[55]

The major objections at first to student assistance rested on the belief that loans were already available through the National Defense Education Act (NDEA) and the AMA's new loan program. The proponents countered by pointing out that the NDEA program was not structured to meet the needs of medical students with their high expenses and the greater length of their training, which require a longer grace period because of their need to complete internship and residency. The major problem with the AMA loan program was its substantially higher interest payments. The Student American Medical Association and the AAMC were on record as favoring the assistance provisions, while the AMA made a last-minute effort to kill the loan program.[56]

In ensuing years, the loan and scholarship programs were reauthorized with changes in interest rates, maximum allowable award levels, and the administration of the program. While quality and equal opportunity were seen as two benefits to be derived from loans and scholarships, this aid has also been perceived as a lever to concurrently influence geographic location and specialty choice.

Well before the HPEA Act of 1963, Congress was aware of the growing reliance of the U.S. medical system on FMGs. The description of a dual system of care—in which low-income areas are served by foreign-trained physicians unable to speak the language and are of questionable competence—is found in congressional documents today as well as twenty years ago. Many hospitals and mental institutions then, as now, functioned only because of FMGs.

To many in Congress, the idea that "the leader of the free world should go out to these countries which are already deficient in this type of highly skilled personnel and bring their doctors into this country by whatever means we do it" was an indication that something was terribly wrong with our capacity to train physicians.[57] This, coupled with the notion of a dual system of care, made strong arguments for expanding the supply of doctors.

Fueling the fire in the late 1960s was the growing pressure exerted by well-qualified, but unsuccessful, U.S. applicants to medical schools. The argument held: "Why should we rely on FMGs when so many well-qualified U.S. students want to go to medical schools?"

Dr. C. H. Willam Ruhe of the AMA has argued that the social forces leading to an influx of FMGs and those who have created a pool of unsuccessful U.S. applicants to medical schools operate independently of one another. "If the size or number of our medical schools could be doubled to accommodate most of the qualified applicants now being turned away," contends Ruhe, "it would probably have little or no effect upon the influx of FMGs—unless we change our immigration laws." The immigration of FMGs reflect a worldwide trend of educated people to move from the underdeveloped countries to more advanced countries.[58]

Despite this line of reasoning, Assistant Secretary for Health, Theodore Cooper, in late 1975, drew the following inferences:

> Increases in the numbers of U.S. graduates and the likely actions of both private and public sectors in addressing the training of graduate physicians, both foreign and domestic educated, may well produce a downward trend in the influx of foreign medical graduates. Our estimates take into account a possible reduction by as much as 40 percent of the FY 1972 level.[59]

From time to time, there has been the criticism that some protagonists have used the foreign medical graduate issue as a rationalization for increased aid to U.S. medical education. While this may be part of the story, the House health subcommittee, for example, declared in 1975 that foreign medical graduates (whose practice patterns generally follow their U.S. counterparts) do not contribute to solving either geographic or maldistribution problems, but only contribute to the deterioration of the quality of U.S. health care.[60] It was the Senate, however, that squarely faced up to the FMG issue by altering the immigration laws restricting the influx of foreign physicians.[61] The measure survived passage through the conference committee and was finally enacted.

A final objective—national licensure standards—is one that is related to the issues of geographic distribution and quality. Senator Kennedy's committee has discussed the issue for several years, but it has been unable to secure support for national uniform licensing standards. Elimination of "the crazy quilt pattern of licensure" among the states, it has been suggested, would lead to greater assurances for the consumer of his physician's competence.[62]

In addition to the role of licensure in quality assurance, there has been a side to the question that is even more germane to a discussion of physician supply. The Senate subcommittee in the past few years has heard testimony from several experts who have been of the opinion that disparate state licensure laws have impeded the interstate mobility of physicians. The main obstacles are separate basic science exams in some states, limitation of recognition of National Board Certificates, failure of some states to recognize the uniform standards of the Federation Licensing Examination (FLEX), specific educational requirements in state laws, problems associated with FMG licensure, and failure of most state boards to require proof of continuing competence on the part of licensees.[63]

While there may be valid reasons for uniform licensing standards, it is not clear how much these changes would affect geographic distribution; there has even been a suggestion that it might aggravate the problem since some of the barriers have existed in areas of the country to which physicians would like to migrate.[64] Furthermore, econometric analysis has suggested that licensure barriers probably have little influence on physician location patterns.[65]

THE FEDERAL VIEW OF THE STATES: CONGRESS

Implicit in the marriage of convenience between the federal government and the medical education sector was the understanding that federal support would not cover the full cost of expansion and operating support. How private resources and state funds were to be integrated with federal monies in terms of long-range planning was seldom made explicit by Congress in the authorizing legislation. Nevertheless, certain assumptions were made regarding shared intergovernmental responsibilities.

The remainder of this chapter will examine these less obvious aspects of congressional decision-making with respect to the perceived role of the states. The examples will be of two types: One will deal with the congressional perspective on expected state performance in the medical education sector; the other with the design of legislative programs in a federal system.

When the federal government contemplates entering an area traditionally reserved by the states, there usually is a determination that the states have been inadequately performing this function. In the present case, Congress had to determine whether state and/or private efforts alone would lead to construction of new medical schools and the expansion of existing ones. Next, Congress has to determine the scale and nature of its intervention. Should it provide a stimulatory influence in the way of seed money or limited emergency funding, or should it assume on-going responsibility for various parts of the system?

During consideration of the legislation in 1962, questions from minority members of the House committee were raised about the need for federal action since more than one-third of the 20 new schools claimed to be needed were already being constructed. The seven new schools in planning or construction were the University of Texas, the University of Connecticut, the University of New Mexico, Brown University, Rhode Island, Rutgers University, New Jersey, Michigan State University, and the University of California at San Diego. The minority members also noted that the AMA reported 18 other potential schools in the discussion stage. "Conceivably a Federal program limited to construction assistance might encourage and hasten favorable decisions in these States," they concluded, "but it would certainly slow down any incentive for raising private funds for the same purpose, and would in fact constitute an unnecessary discrimination against those for which financing has been completed."[66]

It is always a knotty problem to determine what the states and the private sector might have done in the absence of federal aid. On the basis of reports from medical deans, the Surgeon General almost 15 years earlier had anticipated an increase of 1,475 freshman spaces if drawing-board medical schools became reality.[67] Indeed, the period from 1948 to 1960 shows an increase of 1,485 first-year places.[68] Table 3.1 shows that between 1946 and 1963 nine public and two private schools were organized.

There are several imponderables to consider. Had we exhausted by the 1960s the potential for new expanded schools without federal aid? Would the fear of a physician shortage have remained so high without a continuing federal interest? Would schools actually have closed as a result of financial distress? To what extent were schools planned during the 1950s and 1960s operating under the assumption that a federal support was inevitable?

Nonetheless, the general impression left by Congress was one of a constructive federal role. The Assistant Secretary of HEW, Boisfeuillet Jones, in his congressional testimony summarized the role of the federal government: "The Federal Government's role in this situation is a traditional one of making stimulatory grants for action at the state and local level in lieu of direct Federal action."[69]

Table 3.1 Medical Schools Organized Between 1946-63

Medical School	*Year Organized*	*Ownership*
University of California, Irvine	1962	PUB
University of California, Los Angeles	1951	PUB
University of Florida, Gainesville	1956	PUB
University of Miami, School of Medicine	1952	PRI
University of Kentucky, Lexington	1954	PUB
University of Massachusetts, Worcester	1962	PUB
New Jersey Medical School, Newark	1956	PUB
University of New Mexico	1960	PUB
State University of New York, Stony Brook	1962	PUB
University of Puerto Rico, San Juan	1949	PUB
Albert Einstein College of Medicine of Yeshiva University	1955	PRI

Source: Medical Education in the United States: 1975-76, *Journal of the American Medical Association* 27 December 1976. pp. 3061-64.

Congressman Morris Udall of Arizona agreed with this point of view when he described the situation in his and other states: "The problem facing Arizona today is not whether or where a medical school should be established—those decisions have been made—but how to meet this heavy financial burden. I am sure my State is not unique."[70]

Even a wealthy state like California, a recipient of other states' medical graduates, sought federal money to expand local production and decrease its dependence on other states. These sentiments were communicated in a letter to Senator Thomas Kuchel by Clark Kerr, president of the University of California. Kerr explained the financial realities as he saw them:

> The State of California is aware of the problem that confronts us and has done its best to find the necessary funds from current revenues and by issuing bonds. But when we consider other educational needs, and the multitudinous institutions and services which must serve the public welfare, it seems clear that we cannot carry this construction program in the high cost medical field without outside help.[71]

Statements by Udall and Kerr were representative of the thinking on Capitol Hill. To quote the chairman of the House committee: "The testimony in the hearings last year and this year is uncontradicted that new medical schools in sufficient numbers will come into existence only if Federal Aid is made available." Furthermore, based on the experience of other federal matching programs, he expected federal support to serve as a "catalyst" to encourage other sources of support.[72]

There is little evidence to suggest that either state officials or the medical schools were unsettled by the offer of federal money. The only critics were conservatives like senators Barry Goldwater and John Tower.

Did anyone consider the roles of the state and the private sector in the "maintenance of effort?" Surgeon General Luther Terry told Congress:

> Therefore, the stimulus has to come from the State or the community. They have to decide that they want a medical school and are willing to take on the responsibility for operating this and, in turn, what they will obtain from the graduates of that school.[73]

If schools were already in financial crisis, how were they to support more students and new facilities without help from the federal government? In essence, the way the federal policy was designed did not allow for, let alone encourage, the states to plan how expansion could help alleviate problems of access.

Statutorily, the states are treated like a silent partner. Although not referred to explicitly, the states were the most likely source of matching funds—certainly for the public institutions and often as well for the private schools. One of the few acknowledgments of state interest in its medical schools appears in Section 721 of the original law (P.L. 88-129) under "Approval of Applications." It stipulates that the Surgeon General along with his National Advisory Council on Education for Health Professions should take the following into consideration:

> (2) in the case of an applicant in a state which has in existence a State planning agency, or which participates in a regional or other interested planning agency, described in Section 728, the relationship of the application to the construction or training program which is being developed by such agency with respect to such State and, if such agency has reviewed such application, any comment thereon submitted by such agency.[74]

A question to be explored in the next chapter is whether or not these considerations in fact played a role in the awarding of grants.

Could Congress have been more thoughtful about the role of the states in the implementation of the program? One interesting perspective on this question can be gained by taking a closer look at the deliberations on the floor of the House over whether the original legislation was actually a *health* bill or an *education* bill—an important consideration at the time, since federal aid to education in 1963 was a highly volatile issue. Despite protestations by the leadership of the Interstate and Foreign Commerce Committee, some members of the Education and Labor Committee attempted to force consideration of a substitute measure. The sponsor of this substitute bill argued: "In the matter of priority it lets the college and the State commission decide which is of the greatest need. We cannot say that the medical profession is in the greatest need and should be handled separately and apart from all other fields of higher education."[75]

To someone familiar with the HPEA program today, it seems inconceivable that there was ever any doubt as to whether aid to medical schools should be deemed a "health bill." It should be kept in mind, nevertheless, that in many states boards of education (or higher education) allocate money to public and, in some instances, to private medical schools. It is apparent that the education committee in Congress was much more sensitive to intergovernmental relations than its health colleagues. Its substitute measure speaks of allotments to states (rather than to institutions), detailed elaboration of state commissions and plans, federal review and evaluation of state plans, and criteria for determining the federal share.

While all of this may have been a more sensible way of administering funds to medical schools, it was obviously not politically practicable at the time. From the medical schools' point of view, they never would have obtained as much money as through direct federal involvement. From the committee's viewpoint, they were not about to give up control to another, weaker committee or forfeit the chance to do something concrete in the ever-popular, vote-getting area of health.

The course plotted by Congress allowed for minimal intergovernmental interaction. The initiatives were left largely in the hands of the medical schools. Designing the program in this manner had certain consequences for administrative action in implementing the program—the topic to be addressed in the next chapter.

NOTES

1. Stephen P. Strickland, *Politics, Science, and Dread Disease: A Short History of United States Medical Research Policy* (Cambridge, Mass.: Harvard University Press, 1972), pp. 55–74.
2. Elton Rayack, *Professional Power and American Medicine: The Economics of the American Medical Association* (Cleveland: The World Publishing Company, 1967), pp. 90–98.
3. "Congress: In Voting Assistance to Health Professions Education, House Demonstrates Its Folkways," *Science*, 3 May 1963, p. 470.
4. U.S., Congress, Senate, *Congressional Record*, 88th Cong., 1st sess., 1963, vol. 109, pt. 12: 16830.
5. Oscar W. Ewing, *The Nation's Health: A Ten-Year Program* (Washington, D.C.: Federal Security Agency, 1948), p. 47.
6. National Fund for Medical Education, Inc., *Medical Education in the United States*, March 1, 1950.
7. Commission on Financing Higher Education, "Financing Medical Education," Association of American Universities, May 1951, p. 1.
8. President's Commission on the Health Needs of the Nation, *Building America's Health: A Report to the President*, vol. 2 (Washington, D.C.: GPO, 1952), p. 131.
9. U.S., Congress, House Committee on Interstate and Foreign Commerce, *Medical School Inquiry: Staff Report*, 85th Cong., 1st sess. (Washington, D.C.: GPO, 1957), p. vii.
10. Ibid., pp. 39–45.
11. U.S. Congress, House, Committee on Interstate and Foreign Commerce, *Health Professions Educational Assistance*, 87th Cong., 2d sess., 1962, H. Rept. 1489, p. 7.
12. See AAMC prepared statement and supporting document for congressional testimony. U.S., Congress, Senate, Committee on Labor and Public Welfare, *Medical, Dental, and Public Health Teaching Facilities: Hearings Before the Subcommittee on Health*, 88th Cong., 1st sess., 1963, p. 145.
13. American Medical Association, Council on Medical Education and Hospitals, *Money and Medical Schools* (Chicago: AMA, 1962), pp. 76–79.
14. U.S., Congress, House, Committee on Interstate and Foreign Commerce, *Health Professions Educational Assistance Amendments of 1965*, 89th Cong., 1st sess., 1965, H. Rept. 781, p. 19.
15. U.S., Congress, House, *Congressional Record*, 89th Cong., 1st sess., 1965, vol. 111, pt. 17: 22469–70.
16. Ibid., p. 22470.

17. *Report of the National Advisory Commission on Health Manpower*, vol. 1 (Washington, D.C.: GPO, 1967), pp. 24–25.

18. U.S., Congress, House, Committee on Interstate and Foreign Commerce, *Health Professions Educational Assistance Amendments of 1971: Hearings Before the Subcommittee on Public Health and Environment*, 92nd Cong., 1st sess., 1971, p. 539.

19. Carnegie Commission on Higher Education, *Higher Education and the Nation's Health: Policies for Medical and Dental Education* (New York: McGraw-Hill, 1970), p. 43.

20. Grace M. Carter, et al., Federal Manpower Legislation and the Academic Health Centers: An Interim Report (Santa Monica, Ca.: The Rand Corporation, 1974), p. 7.

21. House, *Hearings*, 92d Cong., 1st sess., 1971, pp. 452–53.

22. Senate, *Report*, 93d Cong., 2d sess., 1974, p. 27.

23. U.S., Department of Health, Education, and Welfare, Institute of Medicine, *Costs of Education in the Health Professions*, pts. I and II, DHEW Publication no. (HRA) 74–32, January 1974, p. xix.

24. Ibid., pp. 39–54.

25. U.S., Congress, House, Committee on Interstate and Foreign Commerce, *Health Manpower and Nurse Training—1974: Hearings Before the Subcommittee on Public Health and Environment*, 93d Cong., 2d sess., 1974, p. 287.

26. Senate, *Report*, 93d Cong., 2d sess., 1974, pp. 212–13.

27. U.S., Department of Health, Education, and Welfare, Health Resources Administration, Bureau of Health Manpower, *Selected Information on Health Professions Schools*, part II: *BHM Support by Program, FY: 1965–75* (Bethesda, Md.), p. 2.

28. "Minutes of the AAMC Assembly Meeting," *Journal of Medical Education* (May 1970), p. 510.

29. Information provided by the Association of American Medical Colleges.

30. U.S., Congress, House, Committee on Interstate and Foreign Commerce, *Health Manpower Act of 1975*, 94th Cong., 1st sess., 1975, H. Rept. 266, p. 19.

31. "Health Manpower Act: Aid But Not Comfort for Medical Schools," *Science*, 12 November 1976, p. 703.

32. U.S., Congress, Senate, *Congressional Record*, 88th Cong., 1st sess., 1963, vol. 109, pt. 12: 16829.

33. U.S., Congress, House, *Congressional Record*, 88th Cong., 2d sess., 1964, vol. 110, pt. 16: 21607.

34. U.S., Congress, House, *Congressional Record*, 88th Cong., 1st sess., 1963, vol. 109, pt. 5: 6881.

35. U.S., Congress, House, Committee on Interstate and Foreign Commerce, *Health Professions Educational Assistance*, 99th Cong., 1st sess., 1963, H. Rept. 109, p. 10.

36. Ibid., pp. 10–11.

37. U.S., Congress, House, *Congressional Record*, 88th Cong., 2d sess., 1964, vol. 110, pt. 16: 21606.

38. *Report of the National Advisory Commission on Health Manpower*, Volume 1 (Washington, D.C.: GPO, 1967), p. 37.

39. U.S., Congress, House, Committee on Interstate and Foreign Commerce, *Comprehensive Health Manpower Training Act of 1971*, 92d Cong., 1st sess., 1971, H. Rept. 258, p. 36.

40. U.S., Congress, Senate, Committee on Labor and Public Welfare, *Health Professions Educational Assistance Amendments of 1971*, 92d Cong., 1st sess., 1971, S. Rept., p. 30.

41. Eric Redman, *The Dance of Legislation* (New York: Simon and Schuster, 1973), p. 31.

42. Ibid., p. 33.

43. Carnegie Commission, *Higher Education*, p. 58.

44. U.S., Congress, House, *Comprehensive Health Manpower Training Act of 1971*, 82d Cong., 1st sess., 1971, H. Rept. 258, pp. 33–34.

45. U.S., Department of Health, Education and Welfare, *Towards a Comprehensive Health Policy for the 1970's: A White Paper*, May 1971.

46. "Shortage of Doctors—What's Causing It," *U.S. News and World Report*, 25 March 1963, p. 72.

47. Ewing, *Nation's Health*, p. 41.

48. *Building America's Health*, vol. 7, p. 152.

49. ibid., p. 141.

50. *National Advisory Commission*, p. 14.
51. James E. Bryan, "Favorable House Hearings on Family Practice Bill," *American Family Physician*, December 1970, p. 150.
52. See John P. Bunker, "Surgical Manpower: A Comparison of Operations and Surgeons in the United States and in England and Wales," *New England Journal of Medicine*, 15 January 1970, pp. 135-44; and Charles E. Lewis, "Variations in the Incidence of Surgery," *New England Journal of Medicine*, 16 October 1969, pp. 880–84.
53. Eva D. Cohen, et al., *An Evaluation of Policy Related Research on New and Expanded Roles of Health Workers*, Yale University of Medicine, October 1974.
54. U.S., Congress, House, Committee on Interstate and Foreign Commerce, *Health Professions Educational Assistance*, 88th Cong., 1st sess., 1963, p. 40.
55. Special Message to the Congress on Health and Hospital Care, 9 February, 1961.
56. *Congressional Quarterly Almanac*, vol. 19 (Washington, D.C.: Congressional Quarterly Service, 1963), pp. 216–21.
57. U.S., Congress, House, *Congressional Record*, 88th Cong., 1st sess., 1963, vol. 109, pt. 5: 6826.
58. C. H. William Ruhe, "The Private Sector Can Answer the Need," *Prism*, February 1975, p. 16.
59. U.S., Congress, Senate, Committee on Labor and Public Welfare, *Health Manpower Legislation, 1975: Hearings Before the Subcommittee on Health*, 94th Cong., 1st sess., 1975, p. 990.
60. U.S., Congress, House, Committee on Interstate and Foreign Commerce, *Health Manpower Act of 1975*, 94th Cong., 1st sess., 1975, H. Rept. 266, p. 47.
61. *Congressional Quarterly Almanac*, vol. 32 (Washington, D.C.: Congressional Quarterly Inc., 1976), p. 534.
62. Senate, *Report*, 93d Cong., 2d sess., 1974, pp. 113–43.
63. Ibid., pp. 130–134.
64. U.S., Department of Health, Education, and Welfare, *Report on Licensure and Related Health Personnel Credentialing*, DHEW Publication no. (HSM) 72–11, 1971, p. 43.
65. Donald Yett and Frank Sloan, "Migration Patterns of Recent Medical School Graduates," *Inquiry*, June 1974, pp. 125–42.
66. U.S., Congress, House, Committee on Interstate and Foreign Commerce, *Health Professions Educational Assistance*, 87th Cong., 2d sess., 1962, H. Rept. 1489, p. 66.
67. Surgeon General's Committee on Medical School Grants and Finances, *Financial Status and Needs of Medical Schools*, pt. II (Washington, D.C.: Federal Security Agency, 1951), p. 6.
68. Council on Medical Education, American Medical Association, *Medical Education in the United States 1963–1864* (Chicago: 1964), p. 613.
69. House, *Hearings*, 88th Cong., 1st sess., 1963, p. 66.
70. U.S., Congress, House, *Congressional Record*, 88th Cong., 1st sess., 1963, vol. 109, pt. 5: 6808.
71. Letter to Senator Thomas Kuchel. U.S., Congress, Senate, *Congressional Record*, 88th Cong., 1st sess., 1963, vol. 109, pt. 12: 16843.
72. U.S., Congress, House, *Congressional Record*, 88th Cong., 1st sess., 1963, vol. 109, pt. 5: 6812.
73. House, *Health Professions*, 88th Cong., 1st sess., 1963, p. 69.
74. Public Law 88–129.
75. U.S., Congress, House, *Congressional Record*, 88th Cong., 1st sess., 1963, vol. 109, pt. 5: 6840–1.

4

Executive Leadership and Administrative Implementation

Three broad issues are raised in connection with an inquiry into executive branch politics and health manpower policy. First, it will be necessary to consider the role of the President in placing aid to medical education on the nation's agenda and in White House interactions with the bureaucracy. Next, the role of the bureaucracy in administering the programs Congress enacted must be reviewed. And finally, the implications of federal administration for the states must be assessed.

EXECUTIVE LEADERSHIP

In considering the presidential role in health manpower policy, its subsidiary claims on the President's time and attention must be recognized. Curing the physician shortage is one aspect of a national health program that has been part of the Fair Deal, the New Frontier, the Great Society, and the New Federalism. The President, like Congress, lives a political existence, where ends and means get confused, interest groups apply pressure, bargaining is the order of the day, and priorities often change at a moment's notice.

Harry S. Truman

While the first major federal program for medical education aid came during the Kennedy Administration, Presidents Truman and Eisenhower had positions on the issue. In a special health message in 1945, Truman stated that there were sufficient numbers of physicians, but that they were not located where their services were most needed—especially in rural and semirural areas. Truman believed that since doctors cannot be assigned to these areas, they must be attracted to them by adequate health facilities and economic assurances that they will be paid for their services.[1] Truman linked two pet projects: the hospital construction program, later enacted as the Hill-Burton program, and comprehensive national health insurance. Although it is not clear whether Truman eventually succumbed to the theory of a "doctor shortage," the President eventually adopted the position that the nation urgently needed more physicians.[2] He was, moreover, well aware of the financial strain experienced by the medical schools. "The existing sources of support for medical schools," he told Congress, "require supplementation to sustain the expansion that is needed."[3]

Dwight D. Eisenhower

Truman's Commission on the Health Needs of the Nation completed its report at the end of his tenure. While its recommendations were not forgotten, the new President could hardly be expected to champion a cause like federal aid to medical education, a proposal the AMA had opposed. In fact, just a few weeks after his inauguration, President Dwight D. Eisenhower, addressing the AMA House of Delegates, commented: "I have found in the past few years that I have certain philosophical bonds with doctors." Those bonds involved opposition to anything "socialized" that would lead us to "forsake our traditional system of free enterprise."[4] Speaking about federal aid to medical education, he later remarked: "This is one profession we don't want to get under the dead hand of bureaucracy, I assure you."[5]

Eisenhower became convinced, however, that there was an imbalance in the physician supply:

> The rate at which physicians are being graduated from the nation's medical schools is barely keeping pace with the increase in population. There are serious shortages in such specialized fields as psychiatry, pediatrics, and in physical medicine and rehabilitation.[6]

But Eisenhower could not bring himself to support direct federal aid for medical schools. Rather, he encouraged the "back-door" financing of medical education through expanded biomedical research funding:

> The increase in funds which I have requested for the National Institutes of Health and the National Science Foundation will permit a major increase in trainees and research fellows. The program on construction grants for medical research and teaching facilities also offers the opportunity for medical, dental

and other professional schools to expand their student capacity and provide for the training of more physicians, scientists, dentists and other health workers.[7]

John F. Kennedy

At the end of 1958, candidate John F. Kennedy developed position papers for the campaign ahead. With the help of Theodore Sorensen, the "academic advisory committee" was established to tap the ideas and information from the academic community—primarily the Eastern establishment academic community. Among this group of academic advisors, along with John Kenneth Galbraith and Arthur Schlesinger, was Wilbur J. Cohen, who had been teaching social welfare at the University of Michigan since his departure from HEW in 1956.

After Kennedy's victory, many members of the academic advisory committee were put to work to produce task-force reports to help the new President develop a legislative program. Wilbur Cohen headed the President-elect's task-force on Health and Social Security with an assignment "to review from among the most pressing and significant health and welfare proposals those which should have priority in the initial phase of the new administration."[8]

As Sorensen has pointed out, nearly all of the task-force reports were to varying degrees later reflected in legislation. However, the composition of the new President's program did not wait or depend upon completion of the task-force reports. Other legislative inputs were based on campaign pledges and statements, Democratic and nonpartisan legislation not acted upon by the 86th Congress, expiring laws that needed reauthorization, and finally Budget Bureau briefings on an agency-by-agency, issue-by-issue basis.[9]

President Kennedy summed up his view of the federal role in a special message to Congress in early 1961: "Only a part of the responsibility rests with the federal government. But its powers and resources make its role essential in four areas for improving health care: social insurance, facilities, personnel and research."[10]

It is interesting to note the task-force recommendations regarding the President's program for medical education in light of the legislative proposal. The task force made clear that health manpower goals were part of an overall strategy to achieve the major objective—medical care for the aged. The health manpower proposals contemplated: (a) federal support for maintenance and expansion of educational activities in the health field; and (b) federal aid for the construction of new educational facilities and renovation and expansion of existing facilities for the purpose of increasing the number of persons being trained in these fields.

This proposal was, so to speak, ahead of its time in that it contained features that would not be enacted until years later. Provisions in the original Kennedy proposals of 1961 and 1962 included a ten-year construction program, a scholarship program, cost-of-education grants, and planning grants. By 1963, however, the President was forced to compromise and endorsed the Committee's bill, rather than have his own measures introduced.

Lyndon B. Johnson

"As President there is nothing that I enjoy doing more than coming here to the East Room and signing health bills," said Lyndon Johnson.[11] In fact, it became such a habit that within his first four years of office Lyndon Johnson signed more health bills than all the preceding presidents together.

From the beginning, Johnson realized that, as he put it, "the particular companion of poor health was poverty." Thus poor health became one of the principal enemies in the War on Poverty. Declared Johnson: "The Great Society which we mean to build in America must be a healthy society. I pledge my wholehearted energies to make it that way."[12]

A glimpse of the decision-making process in health manpower policy during the Johnson years has been offered by Dr. Edwin F. Rosinski, former Deputy Assistant Secretary for Health Manpower.[13] Following in the wake of an HEW reorganization, which rapidly diminished the Surgeon General's policy role, the chain of command proceeded from the President to the Secretary to the Assistant Secretary for Health and Scientific Affairs down to one of the deputy assistant secretaries. In developing the President's program, the Deputy Assistant Secretary for Health Manpower was assigned a sub-task force that included two other deputy assistant secretaries—one for Health Legislation; another for Planning and Evaluation.

In its deliberations, the sub-task force was careful to consult with other federal agencies having a stake in Health Manpower. A special effort was made to involve the Bureau of the Budget and a member of the President's staff. Consultations with interest groups like the AAMC and the AMA also figured importantly in the deliberations. And beyond these meetings, the sub-task force members met with "almost every vice-president or provost for health sciences and a number of deans." In this way," said Rosinski, "we attempted to both get ideas and generate support within the subgovernment of health for the policies that were emerging from the discussions." One of the major messages the medical educators wanted to get across was summed up thus: "We don't want federal dollars if it's going to tie our hands. Academic freedom, the rights of faculty, and the rights of students must be preserved at all costs."[14]

After four months of work, the recommendations of the health manpower sub-task force were turned over to the Assistant Secretary for Health and Scientific Affairs, who was himself in charge of the President's overall task force on health. The recommendations traversed up the executive ladder to the President, where they were considered in "political, economic, and other realistic terms," along with the myriad of proposals from other parts of the government. It was then the job of the Deputy Assistant Secretary for Health Manpower to translate policy into concrete legislation and the job of the Deputy Assistant Secretary for Health Legislation to work with Congress in enacting the proposals.

Richard M. Nixon

The problems of a Republican president attempting to formulate health policy in the post-Johnson era proved to be substantial. On one hand, conservatives tend to cut government expenditures and keep the federal role to a minimum. On the other hand, the only way to overcome the inefficiency of the health-care delivery system and control inflation seemed to involve more, not less, government.

President Nixon introduced the nation to the Health Care "Crisis" on 10 July 1969:

> The report that I have received from Secretary Finch and Dr. Egeberg indicates that the problem is much greater than I had realized. We face a massive crisis in the area and unless action is taken, both administratively and legislatively, to meet that crisis within the next 2 to 3 years, we will have a breakdown in our medical care system which could have consequences affecting millions of people throughout this country.[15]

Fear of the breakdown of the health-care system was not the ultimate concern or danger:

> What is ultimately at stake is the pluralistic, independent, voluntary nature of our health care system. We will lose it to pressures for monolithic government-dominated medical care unless we can make that system work for everyone in this nation.[16]

With echoes of the Eisenhower Administration, Mr. Nixon's 1970 State of the Union message set out his credo, his strategy to overcome a situation in which "millions of Americans are forced to go into debt today because the Federal government decided to go into debt yesterday. We must balance our Federal budget so that American families will have a better chance to balance their family budgets."[17]

Faced with a Democratic Congress, Nixon's main remedies for the health-care crisis lay in the strategic use of the veto and impoundment. On 27 January, 1970, the President sent his message to Congress, vetoing HEW appropriations. One of the main targets of this veto was the Hill-Burton program. The President declared that a more pressing need was to fund ambulatory-care facilities—a more efficient alternative to expensive hospital care.[18] In November 1970, Nixon foreshadowed an ever-increasing uneasiness with Congress over impoundment. Although he signed a bill extending authorization of four federal health assistance programs (Regional Medical Program, Comprehensive Health Planning, Health Services Research and Development, and the National Health Surveys and Studies), the President warned: "Now that I have signed this bill, I herewith advise the Congress that in the interest of fiscal responsibility I will limit the appropriation requests under its authorization to the amounts that are later determined to be necessary for carrying out its purpose.[19]

Only a few months before, Congress had tried to limit the President's power to impound health funds. Section 601 of the Medical Facilities Construction and Modernization Amendments of 1970 mandated that funds appropriated for any fiscal year be spent. Vetoing the bill, Nixon claimed that any such measures would significantly restrict presidential options in managing federal expenditures.[20]

In early 1971, Richard Nixon unveiled his National Health Strategy in a Special Message to Congress and said: "Nineteen months ago I said that America's medical system faced a 'massive' crisis. Since that statement was made, that crisis has deepened." He told Congress that in 1960 the federal investment in health was $3.5 billion, which by 1971 had climbed to $21 billion. "We are not getting a full return on our investment," he declared.[21]

Basically, the National Health Strategy consisted of a six-point program covering the following areas: (1) encouragement of health maintenance organizations; (2) special needs of scarcity areas; (3) increase medical manpower; (4) malpractice insurance; (5) research on prevention; and (6) national health insurance.

Health policy-making in the Nixon years perhaps can best be understood by examining his use of high-level staff. Presidential scholars will be analyzing the complex relationship between the President and his staff for years to come. At present, what does seem clear is that the President used his staff to circumvent the bureaucracy, which he abhorred as intensely as Eisenhower did. "When I go to a doctor," Nixon told an AMA convention, "when I am sick, I want him to worry about me and not to be worrying about some form he has to fill out for the Government."[22]

The trend toward greater reliance on a growing White House staff began with Nixon's predecessors, but it reached new heights in his administration—much to the consternation of cabinet officials and bureau chiefs. Elliot Richardson expressed his concern:

> For the foreseeable future there will remain the necessity to fix administrative responsibility for the resolution of issues which cut across health, education, and welfare organizational units. A practical issue of consequence is whether that responsibility is to be fixed with the White House Staff or with a Cabinet officer.[23]

Similar complaints from other members of the Nixon Administration had been voiced. Dr. Robert Q. Marston, for example, who was forced out as director of the National Institutes of Health in 1972, described decisions about the National Cancer Institute budget with such phrases as "came out of the blue" and "considerable surprise to me." One might expect the director of NIH to be the President's principal biomedical research adviser. Yet Marston described the policy process in this fashion:

> I would say that what happened in the past couple of years is that we are no longer making budgetary decisions on scientific matters on the basis of debate or a pushing and shoving between the various voluntary agencies and the

congressional and executive branches. Instead, we now have—with the power of veto and all—a real concentration of decision-making in the executive branch and, for all intents and purposes, at the higher level of the executive branch.[24]

This constrained approach toward policy-making was apparently operative in the formulation of health manpower policy as well. *The National Journal,* in a 1971 article, observed that Nixon's health manpower bill was developed "with strictly limited bureaucratic participation—a trademark of his Administration." Assistant Secretary for Health and Scientific Affairs, Dr. Roger Egeberg, commented that the problem with the bureaucracy from the Administration viewpoint was that it too often falls into "patterns of thinking that apply strictly to their own affairs, not to the total picture."[25]

This "counter-bureaucracy" orientation to policy-making has been detailed by Professor Richard Nathan. The main mechanism employed during Nixon's first term was the "working group," composed of White House staff and borrowed agency personnel. Nathan describes the operation of one of these groups:

> Direct relationships were established between White House staff and agency officials well below the level of the Secretary. Only the most astute Cabinet Member could keep on top of this policy process. The typical decision pattern was one of Consensus—building within the working group, with the lead and arbitrary role assigned to [John] Erlichman, or, in the case of welfare, to [Edward] Morgan as his deputy.[26]

The first-term pattern of attempting to circumvent the bureaucracy with the White House personnel proved very difficult. The second-term strategy was based on the presumption that the President had to get his own men—strictly accountable and loyal to him—into key Cabinet posts. It was at this point that the head of OMB, Casper Weinberger, was appointed Secretary of HEW.[27]

Despite President Nixon's efforts to seek to control the bureaucracy, internal struggles for power and exchanges with Congress continued. Interest group leaders paid friendly visits to agency heads, and vice versa.

While a President has the ability to get the policy machinery in high gear over an issue when it commands his attention, those gears will continue to turn without him. Thus, in the Watergate period, while Congress was beginning to prepare for another reauthorization of health manpower legislation, HEW was ready to proceed with or without strong presidential guidance.

The general orientation of the Nixon Administration was to cut the budget wherever possible. The OMB's disenchantment with the capitation program and HEW's growing uneasiness over the possibility of a surplus of physicians made convenient bedfellows of these two power centers. The two major actors in the network were Paul H. O'Neill, associate director for human resources and community development at OMB and HEW Under Secretary Frank C. Carlucci, a former OMB employee. HEW, with its byzantine power structure, could not maintain a cohesive policy consensus on the issue of capitation reduction—

especially in the face of AAMC's intensive lobbying effort directed at the Health Resources Administration, which operated the program. Although HRA's director pushed the AAMC position of maintaining present capitation levels with no strings attached, the budget decision ultimately was made within the Administration to rechannel much of the capitation support into special project grants, which would give HEW greater control over how the money was spent.[28]

Gerald R. Ford

Compared to the heated debate in Congress over provisions of new health manpower legislation, the Ford Administration remained in the background, coming to the fore occasionally to offer an opinion. The general Administration view initially was to continue the Nixon assault on capitation support. Commenting on the Administration-sponsored bill, which he introduced, Senator Jacob Javits said: "I believe the Administration bill S3584 (HR14930) translates into legislation the health manpower themes of the Office of Management and Budget but fails to meet the health needs of the American people."[29]

As the House was about to vote on another bill at the end of 1974, the House Minority Leader received a letter from HEW Secretary Weinberger, expressing the Administration's dissatisfaction over the committee's final compromise:

> In terms of program implications, the bill (HR17084) reflects the concept of continued reliance upon capitation grant subsidies as a major means of financing health manpower education. HR17084 as modified by the full Commerce Committee does, it is true, somewhat decrease capitation grants in the third year. This again is a step which is useful, but which does not go far enough.[30]

With the appointment of Secretary of HEW, Dr. F. David Matthews, and Dr. Theodore Cooper as Assistant Secretary for Health and Scientific Affairs, a turnabout occurred in the Ford policy toward capitation. For several months Cooper had let it be known that he was uncomfortable about the capitation phase-out that he was expected to defend. In Matthews, Cooper found a sumpathetic ear and a co-advocate. The Secretary, a former university president, was well aware of the budgetary problems medical schools would face with the elimination of capitation payments. He argued that capitation could be a useful tool for pushing the schools to address geographic and specialty distribution. President Ford relented.[31]

Congressional leaders finally managed to maneuver a bill through the Conference Committee and the full House and Senate not long before the 1976 Presidential election. Although several features of the bill—not the least of which was a $1.3 billion authorization level—displeased President Ford, he signed the bill in the face of conflicting advice. Favoring a veto were White House counselors Alan Greenspan and L. William Seidman, the OMB, and the Treasury Department. Despite their own reservations, HEW and the professional interest groups convinced the President that the measure was the best that could be expected in light of the many tough regulatory conditions that had been defeated.[32]

EXECUTIVE AGENCIES AND ADMINISTRATIVE CONTROL

The Congress, the President, and the bureaucracy all have a hand in policy formulation and administration. However, most policies are not self-executing; consequently, structures need to be created or adapted to administer them. While other actors in the governmental system may affect the administration of a program, some organizational entity is usually at the center of the activity.[33] It may be said that the President performs the role of "chief executive," yet as Seidman notes, with few exceptions, "it is the agency heads, not the President, who have the men, money, materiel, and legal powers."

> As a general rule, the President cannot enter into a contract, make a loan or grant, initiate a public works project, or hire and fire Federal employees other than those on his own staff. To work his will in the Congress and outside community, the President must have at his disposal the trade goods controlled by the agencies and be able to enlist the support of their constituencies.[34]

As for Congress, it has provided only limited guidelines to the administration of most programs. In the particular case of health manpower legislation, congressional action in prescribing administrative implementation has taken several forms:

1. Establishing statutory definitions, conditions, and eligibility upon which criteria are based for who is awarded grants.

2. Through the appropriations process, controlling the spigot of funds—not only for grants, but for money to hire personnel to administer the program.

3. Influencing the structure of executive agencies by approving executive reorganization plans, creating new agencies, or establishing formal advisory groups.

The President, using the power of his position, has, parallel with Congress, his own means of influencing administration. He may attempt to intervene in the process of translating Congress' laws into program operation via regulation writing; he will use his budgetary power to influence appropriation levels; and finally he may attempt to restructure the bureaucracy.

TRANSLATING CONGRESSIONAL LANGUAGE AND INTENT

The General Accounting Office (GAO), as Congress' main investigative arm, in two major reports looked into the administration of the HPEA program.[35] In so doing, it touched upon several problems that HEW encountered in its task of operationalizing the congressional mandate.

In evaluating how well an agency performs its tasks, one must compare progress toward achieving the legislative goals. Two of the goals the GAO concentrated upon were alleviating "shortages" and improving "quality."

The authors of the GAO report insisted that the size and importance of the program "make it necessary for NIH to determine, as accurately as practicable, what the shortages are and what personnel would be required to provide a reasonable level of health care for the people of the United States."[36] In essence, HEW's reply could be categorized under the heading "Easier said than done, but we're trying anyway." GAO investigators reported:

> Bureau officials said that they had come up with some goals for the program but that these were based on what the schools planned to do and on the amount of funds available for the program, not on what needed to be done to eliminate shortages of health personnel. They told us that determining these shortages was a very complex undertaking and that it might prove impossible to come up with definitive determinations. They noted that many factors had to be considered, such as population shifts, the ages of practicing professionals, and how to get professionals to locate in areas of need. They noted also that, if the present method of providing health care were changed, it would probably help to alleviate some of the problems of supply.[37]

This illustrates the problems of trying to operationalize a complex concept like "shortages." The tendency, of necessity, will be to take the pragmatic approach as described by the bureau officials.

Another item attacked by the GAO was the question of improved "quality." Reporting on their discussions with HEW officials, the GAO investigators recounted the HEW dilemma:

> NIH told us that educators, particularly in the field of medical education, seemed unable to agree on what constituted quality in education and that, in view of this, NIH did not plan to establish formal criteria for measuring the progress made in improving quality.[38]

The GAO centered its criticism of HEW's management of the special and basic improvement grants on its failure to establish uniform criteria for classifying faculty members as full or part time and the extent to which grant funds may be used for faculty support. Because most schools used their improvement grant awards for faculty salaries, this issue became an important aspect of defining "quality." The GAO believed that Congress had intended the money to be used solely for educational purposes, while HEW argued that it was appropriate to support faculty members regardless of the distribution of effort between teaching and other activities, if that support would prevent closure of a school.[39]

In the area of student assistance, the scholarship program established by Congress created problems of interpretation with the statutory phrase "exceptional financial need." The GAO contended:

> NIH has not provided additional criteria or guidance to the schools concerning how to distinguish exceptional financial need from other need. As a result,

distributions of HSAP scholarship funds often have been based on imprecise or arbitrary criteria resulting in inconsistent and inequitable awards.[40]

HEW admitted that, through lack of adequate personnel to monitor the program, the department was forced to rely on the schools to administer the funds responsibly and adhere to the guidelines. This may be an understatement considering that the GAO discovered such abuses as the medical student who used a $1,000 health profession loan to pay for his girl friend's abortion or the student who used his loan for a summer European tour.[41]

One set of issues causing concern in the past, and likely to continue to do so in the future, relates to attempts to administer programs addressing distribution by geography and by specialty. For instance, what is primary care? Or, how does one define a "shortage" area? The latter problem had to be dealt with in organizing the National Health Service Corps. However, there has been apprehension over any large national effort involving numbers of medical graduates. Such a program is liable to run into difficulties with states that have been trying to address their own maldistribution problems. What may be considered a shortage area in New York may be considerably less serious than a shortage area in Alaska. Will New York medical graduates (be it by carrot or stick) be forced to relocate in Alaska? Perhaps this is an overstatement of the dilemma, but it illustrates the technical and political difficulties that administrative agencies confronted.

The arena of agency regulation-writing came to be seen as a major political battleground. Richard Nixon, at the beginning of his second term, recognized that tighter control of programs required control over regulation writing, grant approval, and budget performance.[42] Congress recognized this, too, as the House Subcommittee on Administrative Law and Governmental Relations considered congressional review of all proposed federal regulations. The AMA, cognizant of the political ramifications, was ready with its own proposed amendments to the Administrative Procedure Act.[43]

THE POLITICS OF FEDERAL SPENDING

Medical schools were eager to participate in the federal largess. For FY 1965, the Department of HEW requested $75 million for construction funds (the total three-year construction authorization being $175 million) for *all* types of health professions schools. Yet, by the beginning of 1964, 70 medical schools and 5 osteopathic schools had already sent leters of intent to HEW. HEW estimated the cost of this requested construction support to be $638 million.[44]

Project grants would be approved on the basis of "relative need," to be determined first by a medical school review panel and then by a national advisory council. To administer the program, HEW initially requested 46 positions. In general, the activities engaged in by HEW personnel were described as "conducting site visits, processing applications, providing technical assistance and consultation to sponsoring agencies or groups, developing guide materials pertaining to the design and functional layout of the health profession schools, maintaining surveillance over manpower needs, and inspecting projects and certifying Federal payments."[45] In five years (1969), the number of permanent positions for HEW's health manpower enterprise totaled 449.[46] By 1973, the total number of positions stood at 851.[47]

Budgeting has been described as "reciprocal expectations that lead to self-fulfilling prophecies."[48] In other words, agency officials expect to have their budget cut, so they pad. The Bureau of the Budget and subsequently the congressional appropriations committees, aware of this strategy, will make the expected cuts. Within the congressional appropriations committees, the House (where appropriation bills originate) has traditionally taken the part of the "heavy," while the Senate is usually expected to restore some of the eliminated funds.

Health Manpower appropriations deviate somewhat from the general pattern, following more closely biomedical research funding, in which the appropriations chairmen, interest groups, and agency officials closely ally themselves against the Bureau of the Budget and the President.[49] The following is a fairly typical exchange between bureaucrat and committee chairman on the subject of health manpower appropriations:

Senator [Listor] Hill. Am I right that the Bureau of the Budget reduced your funds some $35 million for the construction of teaching facilities for medical and dental personnel?

Dr. Graning. Yes, sir.

Senator Hill. That was quite a cut, was it not?

Dr. Graning. Yes, sir.

Senator Hill. Did you ask for the full amount authorized?

Dr. Graning. Yes, sir.

Senator Hill. The cut of $25 million?

Dr. Graning. That is right.

Senator Hill. In other words, instead of getting $185,202,000 such as you requested, this budget allowed you $160,794,000?

Dr. Graning. Yes, sir.

Senator Hill. Do you have more than enough applications for this $25 million?

Dr. Graning. Indeed, we do.

Senator Hill. Are they all good applications?

Dr. Graning. They are. We are very proud of the process that has been established for reviewing these applications. We have excellent cooperation from the leaders in the field of education in the various professional disciplines. We have review committees which consider them very carefully and all projects that have been approved represent excellent educational facilities.

Senator Hill. To help meet the shortage, you are talking about but not meeting it fully, is that right?

Dr. Graning. Yes, sir.

Senator Hill. Thank you very much, Doctor. We appreciate your statements very much.[50]

Warren G. Magnuson, Senator Hill's successor, also proved to be a champion of health manpower, both in his role on the Appropriations Committee and in sponsoring legislation like the National Health Service Corps. In his 1974 book, *How Much for Health?*, Magnuson expresses his views about the "doctor-shortage":

Many people try to become fancy about the physician shortage and hide behind phrases like, "It's only a maldistribution problem, and what we really need is to have the doctors in overserved areas move out to underserved areas." Some people have an even fancier solution; they claim we have an over-supply of such things as neurosurgeons, and all we have to do is to have fewer surgeons and get more doctors to move out to areas like Wrangle, Alaska, or Darrington, Washington (neither community having a physician). The people who live in these towns without a doctor shortage or a physician maldistribution or a preponderance of superspecialists. They are concerned that, when they need medical care, they can't get it. Any way it is looked at, it spells not enough doctors providing services to people who need it.[51]

With these beliefs, the senator continually urged HEW bureaucrats to move quicker to implement new programs and implored them to ask Congress for more money to run them. He persisted even in the face of changing views within HEW over whether a doctor shortage existed.

Some members of the Appropriations Committee even went so far as to coach bureaucrats on how to extract the maximum appropriation from Congress. Senator Alan Bible, for instance, lectured one bureaucrat on the importance of dramatizing one's cause:

I would hope you would relate it [the health manpower problem] to statistics because the mere fact that NIH says this is a great problem does not sell it to the people, but when you say 1940, roughly, there were 120 million people in the United States, there are twice as many more people and we have half as many medical schools, that is something people can understand.[52]

To have the appropriations committees as enthusiastic as they were over a program is, of course, an interest group's dream. Yet the favors the committee can bestow also have their limits, as the AAMC representative Dr. Merlin K. Du Val learned during hearings on FY 1970 appropriations.

Dr. Du Val. If one measures this extraordinary need against the original appropriation authorization of $170 million, it can be seen that even if that amount were available we would still be behind. When this need is measured against the current request of $118.1 million, this leaves us too far behind, with no way to close the gap. . . .

Mr. [Daniel] Flood. If we ever appropriated what Congress authorized for public works, I am sure you will have no idea the number of billions of dollars that would amount to.

Mr. Du Val. Dr. Chapman has already referred to the fact we know each group coming in for appropriations can tell you why it is most important.

Mr. Flood. I was speaking only with reference to the difference between authorizations and appropriations. I repeat, for the purpose of emphasis, if we ever appropriated all the fund authorized on the books today for public works there would not be any money for anything else. Every Congressman has his river and dam and something or other, and the books are filled with authorizations. There is nothing sacred about an authorization.[53]

Dr. Du Val, then a medical school dean, would in a short time learn firsthand as Assistant Secretary for Health and Scientific Affairs the realities of the federal appropriations process.

The general outline of federal spending decisions might be described according to the roles various actors play in the process. The interest groups have always recommended greater authorization levels than the substantive committees have granted in the end. These congressional authorization levels, however, were in excess of what the OMB was likely to approve, and HEW bureaucrats, consequently, would base their calculations and strategies on what they thought the OMB might finally accept. The appropriations committees tended to restore funds cut from the budget by OMB, with the Senate committee generally advancing the cause for higher spending levels. President Nixon attempted to counteract such moves through use of impoundment.

Obviously this process does not lend itself to long-range institutional planning—at least as far as medical school administrators are concerned. Interest groups, however, can play a significant role in smoothing over some of the problems created by the inherent uncertainties. The AAMC, for example, often functions as a communications link between government and its member medical schools. The following item from the AAMC Newsletter illustrates this point:

Delayed consideration of health manpower legislation may result in some fiscal uncertainty for schools planning in advance for the 1975–76 academic year. The availability of federal funds is less uncertain for the fall of 1974. This assessment takes into account the June 30 expiration of present health manpower legislations.[54]

In addition to providing counsel to its members, by participating in appropriations politics, the AAMC has been able to communicate to the government information concerning the administration of federal programs.

While the AAMC represents the interests of the medical education community as a whole, it should also be remembered that some individual medical schools have another form of representation—members of the Appropriations Committee themselves. Let us consider Richard F. Fenno's explanation for why a seat on the Appropriations Committee has been a cherished position:

Any financial resources a Congressman channels into his district must come via contact with an executive agency. And membership on the Appropriations Committee was sought by most members for the power over agency conduct it would bring. In some cases influence with the agencies is tied exclusively to the desire to get things for one's constituents. A senior member summed up his reasons for seeking membership: "It's the Committee that gives you the most power with government agencies; and you're in touch with them all the time for your constituents."[56]

While it is not easy to document systematically how much influence has been applied to the awarding of HPEA grants, medical school administrators have been known to cultivate the good will of congressmen on the appropriations committees.

EXECUTIVE REORGANIZATION

Responsibility for administering the health professions educational assistance programs from the beginning was assigned to the Public Health Service (PHS). Although health manpower has remained within the PHS over the years, the agency itself has undergone several organizational changes—the most significant of which was the diminution of the role of Surgeon General in 1968 from the head of the agency to chief deputy of the new Assistant Secretary for Health and Scientific Affairs. Through the years, health manpower has been a major player in the organization-chart hopscotch inflicted on the Public Health Service.

At first, the HPEA construction program was administered by the Division of Hospital and Medical Facilities, the same agency operating the Hill-Burton health-care facilities construction program. The loan program was administered by the Division of Community Health Services. These two divisions were part of the Bureau of State Services, one of five major branches of the PHS (the other four being the Office of the Surgeon General, National Library of Medicine, Bureau of Medical Services, and the National Institutes of Health).

There was a generalized feeling in the mid-1960s that HEW's programs were fragmented and uncoordinated. Changes in HEW leadership, the publication of a report to the President on the activities of NIH, and the formation of a special House subcommittee to investigate HEW were all portents of impending reorganization. The House subcommittee was particularly interested in HEW's health manpower effort and supported the concept of a Bureau of Health Manpower to overcome a fragmentation in which "training and training facilities construction grants derive from numerous sources; statistical and other manpower data is collected and evaluated in various places; and manpower planning is fragmented among many offices and administrators."[56]

Testifying before the House Committee on Government Operations, which has jurisdiction over reorganization, HEW Secretary John Gardner suggested that the rationale for reorganization was to overhaul the bureau structure in terms of current problems in functional areas of concern.

> The Bureau of Health Manpower will have the primary concern for building an adequate supply of health manpower for the Nation. It will be responsible for projecting manpower needs and programs to meet them. It will serve as a central point of information for educators, administrators, and others involved in the training of professional and subprofessional health workers.[57]

The AAMC applauded the restructuring of the PHS, including the new statutory power of the Secretary to reorganize the Service when and how he deemed appropriate. Commenting on the significance of this measure, AAMC President, John A. D. Cooper, observed that there had been little organized opposition to the reorganization, and that this would not have been the case of a decade earlier. "There is probably considerable validity to the viewpoint," Cooper noted, "that Congressional control over the activities of the Public Health Service were [sic] prompted by fear over the involvement of the federal government in the nation's health care."[58]

The Bureau of Health Manpower's independence was short-lived, for little more than a year later (April 1968), it became part of the National Institutes of Health. By January 1969, its name had been changed to the Bureau of Health Professions Education and Manpower Training and its structure reorganized. One reason offered for the shift to NIH was that Secretary Wilbur Cohen perceived that, under NIH's umbrella, the bureau might have a better chance of increased funding.[59] The official rationale, however, was stated differently:

> Modern biological science and health professions education are so intimately inter-related that their effective and efficient management within this Department requires that they be the responsibility of a single operational unit. This will not be the NIH.[60]

Dr. Robert Q. Marston, NIH head, pointed out that these "efforts to harmonize" would likely be criticized on two counts: namely, that this would further exacerbate the academic community's preoccupation with research as opposed to training, and that research was already enticing young doctors away from the practice of medicine. To the first criticism, Marston replied, in essence, that the problem is not too much research support but too little educational support. To the second criticism, he answered that the number of full-time research physicians is only 1.6 percent of the total, and incomes were considerably higher for those who chose to practice rather than to engage in research.[61]

As part of President Nixon's strategy for controlling domestic affairs, health manpower was now freed from biomedical research and linked with facilities and comprehensive health planning in the Bureau of Health Resources Development. If health manpower was married to NIH in the hopes of increasing its funding, perhaps the converse was intended by divorcing the two in 1973.

What did Nixon's "new federalism" have to do with health manpower? Dr. Kenneth Endicott, director of the Bureau of Health Manpower Education, explained this to the Senate Appropriations Committee: "Implicit in our request is our effort to implement the new federalism, which is being manifested now in general de-emphasis of categorical programs in favor of support through a system of general assistance to the States and revenue sharing."

Senator Warren G. Magnuson challenged Endicott: "You said general assistance to the States. What is that? What is it?"

Dr. Endicott. That would be general revenue sharing.

Senator Magnuson. Well you do not have a revenue-sharing bill. You mean . . .

Dr. Endicott. Specifically in health manpower?

Senator Magnuson. Yes.

Dr. Endicott. No.

Senator Magnuson. Of course you do not.

Dr. Endicott. That would, I assume, be characterized.

Senator Magnuson. We had a revenue-sharing bill which proposes $5 billion, was it not, and there have now been grants made to the States, counties, cities, and what have you, particularly the cities, States, and counties. Well, if you can show me any place where they are using that for health manpower, I would like to see it in the record.

Dr. Endicott. Obviously, I mean the law is permissible.[62]

The AAMC took a dim view of what it considered reorganization for its own sake and pointed out that "no single arrangement ever seems to have been tested long enough to provide an assessment of its efficiency and effectiveness."[63] The AAMC was particularly upset over the separation of NIH and the Bureau of Health Manpower Education. From its perspective of the medical school as a national resource performing indivisible multiple functions, the AAMC saw the separation as a weakening of the "synergism" important in institution building.

With all the changes that have occurred in the wake of decentralization—including the disquietude caused by a protracted fight over reauthorization legislation, reduced funding, further reorganization, and Watergate—it is difficult to test the validity of the AAMC's criticism.

Not long after the 1973 organizational changes, Congressman Daniel Flood asked Assistant Secretary Charles Edwards whether it was time to declare a moratorium on reorganizations. "Somebody," remarked Flood, "is making a career out of them."[64] Edwards was quick to agree.

Nonetheless, another reorganization was in the offing. On 5 May 1975, the Bureau of Health Manpower was established in a realignment of the activities of the former Bureau of Health Resources and Development, many of whose activities were subsumed under the new Bureau of Health Planning and Resources Development. Together, the Bureau of Health Manpwer and the Bureau of Health Planning and Resources Development comprised the two major parts of the Health Resources Administration, one branch of the Public Health Service.

The decentralization of health manpower activities brought about during the Nixon Administration was reversed by Congress in 1977.

Congressional dissatisfaction centered on concern that delegation of obligational authority to the regional offices resulted in a lack of accountability to Congress. As a House committee report noted: "Since the health manpower legislation is national in scope, funds should only be obligated with a view toward national needs.[65] Congress was distressed that certain funds were earmarked as special regional office initiatives. Also, the system for review of applications used by the regional offices was criticized for having lead to approval of grants and contracts of dubious merit.

CONCLUSIONS: IMPLICATIONS FOR THE STATES

Neither President, Congress, nor the bureaucracy is solely responsible for initiating health manpower policies or for implementing them. In passing legislation, Congress is influenced by the President's overall program, his budget, and his philosophy about managing the government. Congress is also sensitive to the bureaucracy, whether representing its own aims or acting as a conduit for interest-group demands. On the other side, the executive branch does not execute legislation without congressional input, a process that has been elucidated in this chapter.

This interplay among federal actors with respect to health manpower policy did not include much direct input from state-level officials as has been typical in many other health policy areas. But then again, the states did not complain loudly about being left out.

For example, in a letter dated 20 August 1965, Paul Rogers, chairman of the House Special Subcommittee on the Investigation of HEW, asked state governors and their health agencies to comment on administrative problems they have had with the Department of Health, Education, and Welfare.[66] A review of the responses to these letters reveals that federal-state relations in aid to medical education were not uppermost in the minds of governors and their health commissioners. In one sense, this is not surprising, since medical education at the state level is usually perceived—at least in terms of organizational responsibility—as an education function, while at the federal level it has primarily been classified as a health issue. On the other hand, with all the rhetoric about health manpower shortages, it seems a bit odd that they did not relate their complaints about older federal programs to the rapidly developing federal presence in medical education.

What were their complaints? Repeated complaints were directed to their necessity of dealing with too many federal agencies, the lack of flexibility in managing project grants as opposed to bloc grants, the difficulty of raising matching funds, the instability of flood-or-famine appropriations, and the lack of state participation in federal policymaking.

One state official who testified characterized the state-federal partnership as one in which the problem was raising "State crops from Federal seed":

The basic point I wish to emphasize during these opening statements is that the responsible persons at the State level are not being sufficiently involved in Federal policy-making, program, writing, and regulation review prior to the "hardening" of such policies and regulations.[67]

There is little indication that states' participation described above was any better, and most likely was worse, in the area of aid to medical education than other areas. While the trend in many intergovernmental projects in the 1960s was purposely to bypass state agencies in favor of local government, the private federalism upon which federal aid to medical education was based had less to do with a conscious decision to bypass states than to adhere to the well-established pattern of a biomedical research funding. There apparently has been little concern over the possible negative effects the money might have on national, state, regional, or local planning. As many local officials observed, the intense pressure to accept federal funds does not permit the luxury of picking and choosing what projects might best serve long-term local needs.

One mechanism for institutionalizing a sensitivity to state needs and planning is through various advisory and review bodies that were established to advise the Secretary on policy matters and to review grant applications. These councils and committees themselves have undergone organizational changes as the health professions educational assistance program grew and as HEW was reorganized. In general, these advisory bodies were composed of HEW Officials, health professions school administrators, and members of the public.

While these committees were supposed to heed state health manpower plans (when they existed), there were several constraints on how attentive they could be to genuine state needs. First, state needs are not easy to define. A large statewide effort is required in order to come to some sort of agreement on needs, together with a workable plan to accomplish goals. Second, the notion that medical schools were resources national, and not local, was widespread. This may have created a certain ambivalence, for instance, in terms of whether the location of a new medical schools was in the best interests of a state. Third, medical schools often had strong influence with weak planning agencies. Pressure on these groups to provide documentation in support of medical school applications was not difficult to secure. Finally, to a great extent, the advisory groups were limited by the external politics of HEW and congressional committees.

The major point to be made is that in private federalism the individual institution is the prime focus—not the state health-care system, and not the state educational system. While it is possible under the best of circumstances to view the institution in the context of these other two systems, the major emphasis is not expended in solving system-wide problems through federal-state cooperation.

State officials are beginning to become aware that they have been left out of the decision-making process. Their assertiveness in contesting certain aspects of 1975 health planning legislation may be a portent of future campaigns. In the implementation of the planning law, they soon discovered that a network of private nonprofit agencies was developing that could potentially undermine the control of state and local public agencies over health resources development. Lobbying efforts were focused on HEW to make favorable decisions with regard to the designation of health services areas. In many respects, these efforts were successful.[68]

Although hardly an exhaustive lobbying campaign, some small efforts have been launched on the health manpower front. For example, the representative from the National Conference of State Legislatures, in testimony before Senator Kennedy's Subcommittee on Health, presented an old dictum of federalism, but one that was hardly ever applied to health manpower. He said: "Federal assistance is perhaps made most meaningful in assisting the States in devising their own answers to the health manpower problem. In this way, a better handle on the problem can be achieved because the resources of the State are more efficiently mobilized."[69]

Do states have the will, power, and the means to devise answers to the health manpower problem, especially when that answer may involve moving complex organizations like medical schools in directions contrary to their own inclinations? Have states shown that they have the capacity to efficiently mobilize their own resources—as well as the federal government's resources—to solve health manpower problems? It is with these questions in mind that we turn to an examination of state politics and the expanding physician supply.

NOTES

1. Special Message to the Congress Recommending a Comprehensive Health Program, 19 November 1945.
2. Annual Message to the Congress on the State of the Union, 9 January, 1952.
3. Message to Congress on the State of the Union and on the Budget for 1947, 21 January 1946.
4. Remarks to the Members of the House of Delegates of the American Medical Association, 14 March 1953.
5. Remarks on Receiving the Frank H. Lahey Award from the National Fund for Medical Education, 16 November 1954.
6. Special Message to the Congress on the Nation's Health Program, 26 January 1956.
7. Ibid., p. 237.
8. Theodore Sorensen, *Kennedy* (New York: Bantam Books, 1965), p. 118.
9. Ibid., p. 237.
10. Special Message to Congress on Health and Hospital Care, 9 February 1961.
11. Remarks on the Signing of the Partnership for Health Amendments of 1967, 5 December 1967.
12. Presidential Policy Paper No. 2: The Nation's Problems of Health, 1 November 1964.
13. Edwin F. Rosinski, "Health Manpower: More Than a Numbers Game," in *Politics of Health*, eds., Douglass Cater and Philip R. Lee (New York: Medcom Press, 1972), pp. 61–74.
14. Ibid., p. 70.
15. Remarks at a Briefing on the nation's Health System, 10 July 1969.
16. Ibid.
17. State of the Union, 22 January 1970.
18. Veto Message on HEW Appropriations, 27 January 1970.

19. Statement on Signing a Bill Extending Authorization of Four Federal Health Assistance Programs, 2 November 1970.

20. Veto of the Medical Facilities Construction and Modernization Amendments of 1970, 22 June 1970.

21. Special Message to Congress Proposing a National Health Strategy, 18 February 1971.

22. Remarks to the AMA's House of Delegates Meeting in Atlantic City, 22 June 1971.

23. Elliot L. Richardson, *Responsibility and Responsiveness: II: The HEW Potential for the Seventies,* 18 January 1973, pp. 7-8.

24. "Too Much Politicking in American Scientific Decisions," *Prism* I (December 1973): 265-69.

25. John K. Iglehart, "Health Report/Administrations Congress Struggle for Solution to Health-Manpower Shortage," *National Journal,* 5 June 1971, p. 1201.

26. Richard Nathan, *The Plot that Failed: Nixon and the Administrative Presidency* (New York: John Wiley and Sons, 1975), pp. 45-46.

27. Ibid., pp. 59-76.

28. John K. Iglehart, "Health Report/Maldistribution of Physicians is Focal Point of Manpower Debate," *National Journal Reports,* 28 December 1974, p. 1952.

29. John K. Iglehart, "Health Report/Kennedy Effort to Revise Health Manpower Carries Over to '75," *National Journal Reports,* 28 December 1974, p. 1952.

30. Ibid.

31. New York *Times,* 6 October 1975, p. 30.

32. John K. Iglehart, "Ford Shuns Advice in Signing New Health Manpower Bill," *National Journal,* 23 October 1976, p. 1513.

33. Charles O. Jones, *An Introduction to the Study of Public Policy* (Belmont, Ca.: Duxbury Press, 1970), p. 93.

34. Harold Seidman, *Politics, Position, and Power: The Dynamics of Federal Organization* (New York: Oxford University Press, 1970), p. 73.

35. U.S., Comptroller General, *Program to Increase Graduates from Health Professions Schools and Improve the Quality of Their Education: Report to the Congress* (Washington D.C.: General Accounting Office, 1972); and *Congressional Objectives of Federal Loans and Scholarships to Health Professions Students Not Being Met* (Washington, D.C.: General Accounting Office, 1974).

36. Comptroller General, *Program to Increase Graduates,* 1972, p. 30.

37. Ibid., p. 30.

38. Ibid., p. 33.

39. Ibid., pp. 35-37, 54-55.

40. Comptroller General, *Congressional Objectives,* 1974, p. 26.

41. Ibid., pp. 8-9.

42. Nathan, *The Plot That Failed,* p. 62.

43. American Medical Association, *Legislative Roundup,* 24 October 1975.

44. U.S., Congress, Senate, Committee on Appropriations, *Labor-Health, Education, and Welfare Appropriations for 1965:* Hearings, 88th Cong., 2d sess., 1964, pp. 38-43.

45. U.S. Congress, Senate, Committee on Appropriations, *Labor-Health, Education, and Welfare Appropriations: Hearings,* 89th Cong., 2d sess., 1966, p. 742.

46. U.S. Congress, Senate, Committee on Appropriations, *Labor-Health, Education, and Welfare Appropriations: Hearings 91st Cong., 1 sess., 1969, p. 1776.*

47. U.S. Congress, Senate, Committee on Appropriations, Departments of Labor and Health, Education, and Welfare and Related Agencies Appropriations: Hearings, 93d Cong., 1st sess., 1973, p. 2166.

48. Aaron Wildavsky, *The Politics of the Budgetary Process,* 2d ed. (Boston: Little, Brown, 1974), p. 23.

49. Ibid., pp. 35, 48.

50. U.S. Congress, Senate, Committee on Appropriations, *Labor-Health, Education, and Welfare Appropriations: Hearings,* 89th Cong., 2d sess., 1966, pp. 742-43.

51. Warren G. Magnuson and Elliot A. Segal, *How Much for Health?* (Washington: Robert B. Luce, Inc., 1974), pp. 147-48.

52. U.S. Congress, Senate, Committee on Appropriations, *Labor-Health, Education, and Welfare Appropriations: Hearings,* 91st Cong., 1 sess., 1969, p. 1855.

53. U.S. Congress, House, Committee on Appropriations, *Labor-Health, Education, and Welfare Appropriations: Hearings,* 91st Cong., 1st sess., 1969, p. 761.

54. Association of American Medical Colleges, *Weekly Report*, no. 54 74–17, 29 April 1974.
55. Richard F. Fenno, Jr., *The Power of the Purse: Appropriations Politics in Congress* (Boston: Little, Brown, 1966), pp. 86–87.
56. U.S. Congress, House, Committee on Interstate and Foreign Commerce, *Investigation of HEW: Report of the Special Subcommittee on Investigation of the Department of Health, Education, and Welfare*, 89th Cong., 2d sess., 1966, p. 83.
57. U.S., Congress, House, Committee on Government Operations, *Reorganization Plan No. 3 of 1966 (Public Health Service)*, 89th Cong., 2d sess., 1966, p. 9.
58. John A. D. Cooper, "A New Look at the Public Health Service," *Journal of Medical Education* 41 (August 1966): 804.
59. Rufus E. Miles, Jr., *The Department of Health, Education and Welfare* (New York: Praeger, 1974), p. 216.
60. U.S., Congress, Senate, Committee on Appropriations, *Labor-Health, Education, and Welfare Appropriations: Hearings*, 91st Cong., 1st sess., 1969, p. 1020.
61. Ibid., p. 1021.
62. Senate, *Appropriations Hearings*, 93d Cong., 1st sess., 1973, p. 2118.
63. U.S., Congress, House, Committee on Interstate and Foreign Commerce, *Reorganization of Health Programs in HEW: Hearings Before the Subcommittee on Public Health and Environment*, 93d Cong., 1st sess., 1973, p. 132.
64. U.S., Congress, House, Committee on Appropriations, *Labor-Health, Education, and Welfare Appropriations: Hearings*, 93d Cong., 2d sess., 1974, pp. 8–9.
65. U.S., Congress, House, Committee on Interstate and Foreign Commerce, *Health Manpower Act of 1975*, 94th Cong., 1st sess., 1975, H. Report 266, pp. 68–69.
66. U.S., Congress, House, Committee on Interstate and Foreign Commerce, *Investigation of HEW: Hearings Before the Special Subcommittee on the Investigation of the Department of Health, Education, and Welfare*, 89th Cong., 1st sess., 1966.
67. Ibid., p. 252.
68. John K. Iglehart, "Health Report/States, Cities Seek Role Over Regional Planning Bodies," *National Journal*, 23 August 1975, p. 1207.
69. U.S., Congress, Senate, Committee on Labor and Public Welfare, *Health Manpower Legislation: Hearings Before the Subcommittee on Health*, 94th Cong., 1st sess., 1975.

5

Illinois: A Case Study

Whether through lack of resources, incompetency, or disinterest, the states, in the federal view, had done little to deal with the physician-shortage problem. Therefore, it was up to the federal government to go to the heart of the production process—the medical schools.

This approach raises the question whether private federalism is an effective way of solving problems that have both a national and local dimension. If circumstances warranted the federal government bypassing the states to deal directly with medical schools, it is important to learn what negative impacts resulted and how they might be avoided in future programs.

In shifting attention from federal policy-making to state activity, the following questions will serve to guide the following case study in revealing the nature of the three-cornered relationship:

What did states seek to accomplish?

How did they formulate and implement their plans?

To what extent did states plan with an eye to federal aid, and how did federal dollars ultimately impact state planning?

What areas of potential complementarity might have been developed between the federal government and the states?

This chapter and the next present details of one state—Illinois—in search for answers to these questions. Following is a chapter that takes a more macroscopic view in an effort to generalize the Illinois experience.

In light of the conventional wisdom of the 1960s—that the nation was suffering a "doctor shortage"—one takes as given that the objective of state policy-makers was to increase the physician supply. A second broad objective was to increase opportunities for state residents to attend medical school. In most cases, states sought to achieve both objectives simultaneously through policies of expanding institutions—both public and private—that provided medical education. These policies were responsive to both objectives, because expanding medical education capacity provided more opportunity for residents to pursue medical training; it also promised to enlarge the supply of physicians for the state, on the assumption that graduates would practice where they were trained. While this approach could be challenged as not the most cost-effective means of meeting a state's health-care delivery needs, most state officials and interest groups were comfortable with it.

This case study explores how Illinois pursued the goal of expanding medical education in the context of a changing federal role. The study begins with a review of how state government came to take action, followed by the administrative and budgetary politics involved in the implementation. Next, since local governments are also concerned about the local supply of physicians and since the presence of a medical school can have a significant impact on a community, the local role as distinct from the state role is reviewed. The final section explores the issue of federal influence on the state.

THE DECISION TO EXPAND

During the late 1960s, Illinois embarked upon an effort to increase its health manpower supply. The vehicle for state action was a study commissioned by the Illinois Board of Higher Education.[1] Having adopted the report, the public agency oversaw the implementation of its recommendations—at times to the consternation of professional interest groups.

The confluence of state and federal funds flowing into health professions education had a major impact on the physician supply in Illinois. Between 1966–67 and 1974–75, Illinois medical schools increased their *first-year* enrollments from 575 to 1,013. This was accomplished in part by the creation of the two new schools—University and Southern Illinois University (Table 5.1). Tables 5.2 and 5.3 display projected enrollments and numbers graduated.

Not only did the state commit itself to supporting the additional students in its public universities, as well as providing generous capitation support for Illinois residents in private institutions, but it also agreed to make grants to affiliated hospitals. Between FY 1972 and FY 1976, the state appropriated $137.5 million for operations and grants in its health education programs (medicine, dentistry, nursing, veterinary medicine, and allied health). Almost three-fourths of this money, nearly $100 million, was devoted to supporting medical education. In addition, by FY 1976, the state had appropriated $100 million for capital

Table 5.1. First-Year Enrollments in Illinois Medical Schools, 1966-67 and 1974-75 by Type of Control

School	1966-67	1974-75
	(numbers enrolled)	
Private		
Chicago Medical School	75	107
Northwestern University	138	173
Loyola University (Stritch)	89	136
University of Chicago (Pritzker)	73	106
Rush University	—	90
Total private school enrollment	375	612
Public		
University of Illinois	200	341
Southern Illinois University	—	60
Total public school enrollment	200	401
TOTAL	575	1,013

Source: "Medical Education in the United States: 1966-67," *Journal of the American Medical Association*, 20 November 1967; "Medical Education in the United States: 1974-75," *Journal of the American Medical Association*, 29 December 1975.

projects for the public medical schools, including almost $60 million for a new University of Illinois teaching hospital.[2]

One might wonder why a state that had a history of losing to other states almost three-fourths of its medical school graduates would wish to invest so many resources in expansion. Urbanologist Pierre DeVise, who has analyzed physician migration patterns in Illinois over many years, has queried what state decision-makers had hoped to accomplish. DeVise views the state medical education plan as nothing less than "a subsidy for California-bound physicians attracted by the lures of climate, glamour, and federal dollars."[3]

Seemingly this would suggest that states do not have the capacity to allocate resources to their best advantage. But further analysis is required. The answer to the question of whether states can plan lies at the nexus of the health-care system, the education system, and the political system, and this must be explored more carefully.

EARLY STUDIES

Prior to the decision of the Illinois Board of Higher Education to promote a massive health education expansion, the question of whether Illinois had an adequate supply of doctors was periodically addressed. The issue was usually approached in the context of higher education policy rather than as part of health policy per se. For example, in 1943, the General Assembly created the Commission to Survey Higher Educa-

Table 5.2. Projected Enrollments in Illinois Medical Schools

	1975-76		1976-77		1977-78		1978-79		1979-80	
	Illinois Resident	*Total*	*Illinois Resident*	*Total*	*Illinois Resident*	*Total*	*Illinois Resident*	*Total*	*Illinois Resident*	*Total*
Chicago Medical School/UHS	219	396	212[b]	332[b]	228	350	237	365	243	375
Loyola University	246	394	249	390	246	390	246	390	246	390
Northwestern University	350	707	361	707	364	707	364	704	364	704
Rush University	260	312	288	345	359	428	390	456	385	460
Southern Illinois University	171	171	212	212	252	252	276	276	288	288
University of Chicago	161	414	168	400	168	400	168	400	168	400
University of Illinois	1,296[a]	1,322	1,447	1,477	1,617[a]	1,649	1,752[a]	1,787	1,857[a]	1,894
Chicago	(972)[a]	(992)	(1,028)[a]	(1,049)	(1,099)[a]	(1,121)	(1,146)[a]	(1,169)	(1,201)[a]	(1,226)
Peoria	(118)[a]	(120)	(137)[a]	(140)	(172)[a]	(175)	(206)[a]	(210)	(221)[a]	(225)
Rockford	(108)[a]	(110)	(137)[a]	(140)	(181)[a]	(185)	(206)[a]	(210)	(221)[a]	(225)
Urbana/Champaign[c]	(98)[a]	(100)	(145)[a]	(148)	(165)[a]	(168)	(194)[a]	(198)	(214)[a]	(218)
Total	2,703	3,716	2,937	3,863	3,234	4,176	3,433	4,378	3,551	4,511

[a]Estimated at 98 percent of total.

[b]Decline from previous year because of change in curriculum length.

[c]Figures shown are based on a proposed new clinical school.

Source: "Health Education Commission Recommendations on Medical Education for State of Illinois," Illinois Board of Higher Education, 1 July 1975.

Table 5.3. Graduates from Illinois Medical Schools from 1967-68 to 1973-74

	1967-68		*1968-69*		*1969-70*		*1970-71*		*1971-72*		*1972-73*		*1973-74*	
	Illinois Resident	*Total*	*Illinois Resident*	*Total*	*Illinois Resident*	*Total*	*Illinois Resident*	*Total*	*Illinois Resident*	*Total*	*Illinois Resident*	*Total*	*Illinois Resident*	*Total*
Chicago Medical School/UHS	11	73	17	68	8	70	38	71	42	78	26	82	39	90
Loyola University	49	82	49	86	40	82	61	106	69	103	62	105	73	125
Northwestern University	56	136	48	137	47	143	52	146	44	140	48	146	63	159
Rush University	—	—	—	—	—	—	—	—	—	—	10	32	36	60
Southern Illinois University	—	—	—	—	—	—	—	—	—	—	—	—	—	—
University of Chicago	18	69	22	68	22	62	18	67	25	73	30	84	34	89
University of Illinois	185	186	191	193	193	194	187	189	201	202	211	214	224	227
Totals	319	546	327	552	310	551	356	579	381	596	387	663	469	750

Source: "Health Education Commission Recommendations on Medical Education for State of Illinois," Illinois Board of Higher Education, 1 July 1975.

tional Facilities in Illinois. The Commission report noted that Illinois was doing more than its share to train physicians, since Illinois medical schools enrolled about 1,500 more students from other states than other states who admitted students from Illinois. The authors concluded that no definitive answer could be given to the question whether Illinois had an adequate supply of physicians, except to say that the state compared favorably with its neighbors.[4]

A study by Edward F. Potthoff in 1959 focused on the problem of retraining medical graduates within the state. Unable to attract or retain young physicians, the state, until 1950, had depended upon licensing high proportions of graduates of unapproved or extinct medical colleges (27.2 percent of the supply in 1950); then it turned to foreign medical graduates. Potthoff's solution to the problem of retention was to improve Illinois hospitals' capacity to train interns and residents, rather than to increase opportunities for undergraduate medical training.[5]

Two years later, a report recommending a state plan for public higher education reiterated the need to retain Illinois medical graduates, but it also raised the possibility of establishing a new medical school within the State University system. Increasing enrollment at the University of Illinois College of Medicine was specifically ruled out.[6]

These early studies indicate some awareness at a state level of a problem with a large outmigration of Illinois medical graduates but not serious concern over medical school output. At the federal level, fear of a physician deficit had been escalating during the 1950s and heightened with the publication of the Bayne-Jones and Bane reports.[7] Rosemary Stevens, commenting on this period, noted:

> While it could just as well be argued that there had been too *many* physicians in 1950, or that physician productivity had increased sufficiently to make increasing the numbers of physicians less important, the findings were politically persuasive. In a context of anxiety that American youth were less scientifically proficient than their Russian counterparts, and in mounting interest in the social provision of health services, there were few who were likely to cavil over the need for more rather than less physicians.[8]

It was not until after the Congress passed the Health Profession Educational Assistance Act in 1963 that the enthusiasm on a national level began to be transmitted to the state government. The master planning activities in which the powerful Illinois Board of Higher Education was engaged served as a mechanism to channel the activities of those most anxious to increase the physician supply.

MASTER PLANNING AND HEALTH EDUCATION: THE ROLE OF THE IBHE

In a 1968 report, Robert H. Salisbury assessed the performance of the Illinois Board of Higher Education (IBHE) since its creation by the General Assembly in 1961. He concluded:

"The key word is *system*, for what the board has done is to transform a collection of institutions with different governing boards, geographically specialized interests, and uncoordinated catch-as-can budgeting and appropriations into a state system with explicit criteria and well-developed data to shape decisions.[9]

By virtue of its statutory responsibilities combined with prudent leadership, the IBHE had emerged as a powerful force in state higher education policy-making. Legally, the board is responsible for developing a master plan for higher education, reviewing capital and operating budgets of the institutions for the purpose of making recommendations to the governor and the General Assembly, and approving proposed new programs of instruction, research, and service. The responsibility to advise on budgetary matters has developed into "effective power to coordinate and adjust higher education budgets as to both total amounts and proportionate shares allocated to the various components of the system." Salisbury attributes the early success of the IBHE to its role in taking the Legislature and the governor "off the hook" by making all the tough decisions on priorities and interinstitutional allocations. In addition, its decisions to expand higher education in Chicago proved to be a popular move. It has also gained credibility in the area of cost containment; and both the acknowledged quality of staff and appointed members have added greatly to the prestige of the agency.[10]

Although its initial efforts at creating a master plan did not include consideration of professional education in health, the IBHE recognized the need to deal with this area in its 1964 report:

In the Development of the Master Plan, the Board and its staff were unable to devote the time and money necessary to conduct a study of the needs for new programs in the medical sciences. These needs should be studied by nationally recognized specialists, including representatives from medical schools of several sizes and emphases. Several of the Study and Advisory Committees and both the University of Illinois and Southern Illinois University consider an immediate study essential, especially in view of the new federal monies which will be available for construction of medical facilities.[11]

In its 1965 session, the Illinois General Assembly transformed this recommendation into law directing the IBHE to conduct a comprehensive study to determine state needs for additional programs in higher education for the health professions. The study was to include "the determination of the proper geographic locations for, the probable cost of, and the necessary ancillary facilities such as hospitals and nursing schools required with the establishment of such additional programs, as recommended in the Board's Master Plan."[12]

By March 1966, the IBHE had selected Dr. James Campbell, president of Presbyterian—St. Luke's Hospital, to serve as planning director of the study, by then called "Education in the Health Fields," but now most commonly remembered as the Campbell Report. Dr. W. Randolph Tucker, also of Presbyterian-St. Luke's, was appointed research director.

Financial support for the study came from the board's own resources, private donations, and a special appropriation from the General

Assembly. The latter state funds were contingent upon matching nonstate money, most of which was obtained from Federal Comprehensive Health Planning grants.[13]

The twenty-month study resulted in a two-volume report issued in June 1968. The success of the report can at least in part be credited to a scrupulous concern for legitimacy. One kind of legitimacy was achieved by ammassing a substantial body of data. Three major surveys were undertaken:

1. A representative sample of the general population, classed as consumers of health care, was interviewed about its patterns of health care.

2. Parallel samples of purveyors—physicians, dentists, pharmacists, and hospital administrators—were surveyed, as well as health departments and a group of influential citizens throughout the state.

3. Alumni of the medical schools in Illinois from the classes of 1954, 1955, 1956, 1958, and 1960 were asked about the kinds of medical work they were doing, why they left Illinois or stayed in the state, and what might cause them to return if they had left.

Also, by broadening the base of the study group through the use of advisory committees representing major interests in the state, creditability was further extended and potential criticism averted. The advisory committees were organized along the following lines:

a) A State Advisory Committee, composed of representatives of all the major health fields, as well as representatives from the citizenry at large and appropriate organizations throughout the state, met on three occasions in Chicago. The deans of the five medical schools in Chicago were appointed as an adjunct to aid in the work of this committee.

b) A National Advisory Committee, consisting of outstanding leaders in education in the health fields, met on one occasion in Chicago to consider the postulates and principles upon which this report is based.

c) A Research advisory Committee, composed of representatives of various disciplines, aided in the planning and carrying out of the surveys upon which this report is based. In addition, numerous consultants were held with individual members of this Committee in various cities in the United States.

Individual institutions were also asked to submit reports outlining their future directions in educating health professionals. The University of Illinois, for example, decided to take this opportunity to reassess its institutional goals.[14]

THE CAMPBELL REPORT

Based on the personal health surveys undertaken for the report, it was found that 10 percent of the state's population was without "a regular source of medical care," and an estimated 20 to 25 percent did not have preventive medical-care services. While the ratio of physicians to population in Illinois (133.5 per 100,000) was slightly below the national figure (139.6 per 100,000), the study group found the following regional variations within the state: Southern Illinois had a ratio of 72, Central Illinois a ratio of 88.5, Northwestern 84.8, and Northeastern Illinois-Metropolitan Chicago 162.3. Sparsely populated rural and inner city areas were noted as having especially low ratios.

The major thrust of the recommendation for the medical education sector involved rapid, efficient, and inexpensive expansion using existing programs and facilities wherever possible. The rationale presented was that for one-half of the time and one-fourth of the cost of a new school with new clinical facilities, an existing institution could be expanded. The prescription for expansion along these lines entailed using university graduate programs in the basic medical sciences as a means of enlarging the capacity of schools to handle more students, encouraging private universities to increase their enrollments with the assistance of public monies, establishing new relationships between community hospitals and medical schools, and inducing schools to adopt streamlined and innovative curricula.

Several recommendations were put forward specifically for the University of Illinois and Southern Illinois University. The University of Illinois Medical College was to graduate an additional 200 students annually by augmenting its basic science teaching capability with courses at its sister campuses in Chicago and Urbana/Champaign and by developing clinical centers via affiliations with facilities in Chicago, Peoria, and Rockford, and possibly Champaign/Urbana or Decatur. Southern Illinois University was to establish an innovative medical curriculum capable of graduating 50 students, who would receive their basic training at the Carbondale campus and clinical training in Springfield.

The goal for private medical school expansion was set at an increase of at least 150 graduates annually by the year 1978. To support this growth, the private schools could qualify for single, nonrecurring grants for planning and capital construction, as well as capitation support for their Illinois residents on a formula basis.

Thus for capital construction, schools could obtain $50,000 for each of the first 20 additional Illinois residents accepted and $20,000 for each student beyond 20. On an annual basis, schools would be allowed $6,000 for each additional Illinois resident (a minimum requirement of 20 additional Illinois residents), plus annual stabilization grants that were projected as follows:

School	*Total Number of Illinois Residents Enrolled*	*Amount of Grant*
Loyola University (Stritch)	208	$208,000
Northwestern	217	217,000
University of Chicago (Pritzker)	91	91,000
Chicago Medical School	51	51,000

Surveys of Illinois medical alumni had revealed that only 30.6 percent of the graduates in the years studied remained within the state. Perceiving location of internship and residency as an important influence in ultimate practice site (45.8 percent of the alumni remained in the states where they took their residency), the study group produced a series of recommendations designed "to enhance the educational climate of the State." This was to be accomplished by strengthening and expanding house officer programs throughout the state with the help of funds appropriated to the Board of Higher Education. The emphasis was to be on confederated networks of medical school affiliated hospitals—the linkages to be approved by the board. Another strategy centered on improving the state's retention rate by means of a medical student loan program with a service payback provision.

To summarize, the Campbell Report had something for everyone who was anyone in the health profession education system. But could the state afford to play the rich uncle? The organization of a Health Education Commission under the IBHE was recommended ostensibly to assist the board in implementing the recommendations of the report—a task that no doubt would require a good deal of political skill.

ADMINISTRATIVE AND BUDGETARY POLICIES

The Health Education Commission

The Health Education Commission, as originally conceived by Campbell and his associates, was to have more autonomy than the organization that finally emerged. Established on 10 September 1968, the HEC's function and membership were described as follows:

> This commission is to be composed of not more than twelve nor less than six members plus a Chairman, all appointed by the Board of Higher Education.
>
> Specific functions of the Commission are to advise on licensing and accreditation procedures for health care workers; report on the implications of health manpower situations for the state's education programs; review all programs seeking state funds through the Board of Higher Education for education in the health fields; advise the Board on requests for, and allocation formula or otherwise of providing continuing state aid to non-public medical and dental schools; and advise the Board upon all other aspects of education in the health fields which in the judgment of the Commission appear to require action.
>
> This Commission is composed of
>
> a) Five individuals with academic or professional affiliations who are knowledgeable on health care education.
>
> b) Five citizens at large who are not directly associated with any institution, organization, or profession dealing with health services or health education and,
>
> c) Three out-of-state consultants with broad knowledge in health education.
>
> A position of Higher Education Medical Officer is created on the Board of Higher Education staff in order to serve the Health Education Commission.[15]

The leadership of the Board of Higher Education shrewdly foresaw the real possibility of the HEC developing into an autonomous body along the same route the board itself had traveled.

The Chairman of the Board, George L. Clements, made it clear from the first that he was not about to delegate his agency's legally assigned functions to the commission. Almost every aspect of the commission's functioning—staffing, employment conditions, operating budget, contracting, office space, and commission membership—was to be subject to board approval and oversight. Above all, the chairman of the commission held office at the discretion of the board.[16]

Despite these early precautions, some members of the HEC believed that the commission should take on an independent advocacy role by appealing directly to the General Assembly and governor to restore budget cuts approved by the board. It did not take long for these organizational relationships to be tested. The commission members were appointed in June 1969, and by the start of 1970 they were to present their recommendations to the board for FY 1971. Translating the Campbell Report recommendations into a budget request, the HEC arrived at a sum of $17,283,827 for medicine, nursing, dental, and allied health programs. The request was based on formula grants for capital, operational, and stabilization purposes.[17]

In January, however, the board had received word from both the General Assembly and the governor that appropriations would be tight. Governor Richard B. Ogilvie, in a letter to the board, wrote:

> The Board of Higher Education has primary responsibility for the allocation of funds within higher education and should make every effort to meet the general guidelines I have conveyed to other state agencies.... In FY 71, higher education must expect to hold the line in aggregate dollar terms at the level of FY 70.[18]

Typical of its position, the board expressed its deep concern about the impact this would have on higher education in Illinois, but it reiterated its resolve to fulfill its responsibility for recommending priorities within the available resources.

The HEC's budgetary recommendations were then reviewed by the board's staff in light of the governor's request to "hold the line." The original figure, in excess of $17 million, was cut to $8 million—45 percent of the requested funds remained for capital and operating expenses at the public institutions and 46 percent for private schools.[19]

At the February meeting, the discussion focused on the propiety of submitting a supplemental budget for the Health Education Commission. Dr. Tucker, representing the HEC, made a case for the need to fund fully the original request and indicated that the "Health Education Commission recommendations would not change." Nevertheless, the board finally voted to accept its staff recommendations of $8 million but agreed to explore the possibility of a supplemental budget with the HEC and the individual institutions.[20]

The discussions culminated in a proposal to submit supplemental appropriation bills separately on behalf of each public institution and one for the private institutions—a tactic that did not succeed. In the midst of this pulling and hauling, significant organizational pressures were mounting to alter the role of the HEC in relation to the board.

Earlier that year, Chairman of the IBHE, George L. Clements, had expressed his displeasure to the Chairman of HEC, Harold H. Hines, Jr., over an incident in which a separate appeal to the Bureau of the Budget had been made by a HEC member attempting to restore budget cuts. Indicating he had the support of the governor, Clements reaffirmed the position that planning for health education could not be divorced from higher education:

> I have nothing but admiration for what has been accomplished in the health education area to date but understandably it has developed into a semiautonomous and independent activity in the total planning and programming of higher education with which the Board of Higher Education is charged.[21]

By June, the board decided to reconstitute the commission and replaced several of the members with nonprofessionals. It also stripped the commission of its own professional staff. The commission members responded with a statement declaring: "The current staff of the Board of Higher Education does not have the experience or the expertise to furnish the kinds of questions and information which are necessary for decisions in the various professional areas." In a separate statement, Dr. Homer M. Kimmich charged that the replacements were "so obviously purely political":

> The Board of Higher Education has made sure through this ploy that dissent to its own uninformed policies is squelched. Having been a major force in U.S. Health Education development in the last half decade, the Health Education Commission will now almost certainly assume a secondary role in planning.[22]

Whether or not this prophecy has been fulfilled is unclear. Certainly, the wildest dreams of medical education expansionists have failed to become reality, but neither has medical education been drastically cut back. Rather than saying the HEC has taken a secondary role in planning, it is probably closer to the truth to say that it became an effective extension of its parent body, using much the same strategy.

This strategy was described by another IBHE Chairman, Donald Prince: "This Board must try to find that delicate balance of the minimum money necessary to support a maximum quality education—and within that balance, must further recommend the complex mixture of allocations to nourish all diverse constituencies of higher education.[23] This philosophy could easily mean nothing more than "it's our job to make everyone happy," if it was not backed up by thorough homework and a leadership that was sensitive to the positions of major actors and adept at persuasion.

Similarly the HEC has carefully recognized the desires of medical schools but also is as equally attuned to the political pressures on the Board of Higher Education. It serves the board by providing legitimacy to budgetary decisions affecting medical education through a visible

Table 5.4. Higher Education Operating Budgets (in thousands of dollars)

	FY 1974 Appropriation	*Institution and Agency Requests*	*BHE Recommendation*	*Governor's Budget*	*Differences between BHE's and Governor's Budget*
Universities	434,968.2	506,326.0	468,228.4	467,213.4	–1,015.0
Community colleges	75,167.7	88,864.1	80,362.5	80,362.6	—
Illinois State Scholarship Commission	65,099.5	74,139.0	75,100.0	73,785.0	–1,315.0
Health Services Grants Act (aid to private health profession's schools)	15,665.0	16,612.0	16,612.0	16,612.0	—
Financial assistance for nonpublic higher education	6,000.0	11,200.0	6,000.0	6,000.0	—
Higher Education Cooperation Act	350.0	2,000.0	800.0	600.0	–200.0
Mid-Illinois Computer Center	—	360.0	312.0	312.0	—
Board of Higher Education	1,043.9	1,120.9	1,120.9	1,120.9	—
Retirement contributions	19,720.0	82,673.6	24,485.5	24,485.5	—
Division of Services to Crippled Children (Univ. of Illinois)	4,315.3	5,226.8	4,315.3	4,615.3	+300.0
Total	622,329.6	788,522.4	677,336.6	675,106.7	–2,230.0
General revenue funds	559,442.8	723,876.3	605,001.6	507,818.6	+2,817.0
University Income Fund	60,928.8	61,246.1	58,935.0	63,888.0	–5,047.0
Federal State Scholarship Incentive Grant	—	1,300.0	1,300.0	1,300.0	—
Other appropriated funds	1,958.0	2,100.0	2,100.0	2,100.0	—

Source: Illinois Board of Higher Education.

process of public deliberation. In return, the board has accepted most of the HEC's recommendations.

Its critics contend that the IBHE is nothing more than an arm of the Bureau of the Budget. If anything, the IBHE posture has been disarming to both the executive and legislative branches. One IBHE chairman, Cameron West, put it this way:

> Here is our best judgment as to the realistic needs of higher education, and a method of funding these needs. If these branches of government disagree on the funding proposal, they can suggest another approach. If they disagree on the level of services recommended, this Board is prepared to recommend what is to be put back.[24]

The challenge is not one that any budget agency or legislative official with a limited professional staff is likely to accpet, nor have they, as Table 5.4 illustrates.

Above all, though, the IBHE has succeeded in minimizing interinstitutional conflict. "The danger lies in internecine warfare, both within the public sector and between the public and private sector," observed West. "If Illinois higher education presents a selfish and quarrelsome image regarding budgets, it will have to expect that others outside higher education will determine its needs and priorities."[25] The alternative—individual institutions lobbying various parts of the government—may have resulted in larger sums of money for favored projects but less stable funding, less rational planning, and probably more arbitrary government interference in institutional development.

Not long after the organizational upheaval of the HEC, Governor Daniel Walker was elected, taking office in January 1973. He appointed as his coordinator for health Dr. Mark Lepper, dean of Rush Medical School. Lepper along with James Campbell, who was president of the then University of Illinois-affiliated Presbyterian-St. Luke's Hospital, were among the major engineers of the subsequent split between the hospital and the University of Illinois—a split that resulted in the organization of the Rush-Presbyterian St. Luke's Medical Center. Needless to say, such a move was not without its tensions. A visitor to either medical school campus would be struck by the uncomfortable geographic proximity of the two institutions, the buildings situated almost like fingers in clasped hands.

Lepper had different expectations of the HEC than what were realized; he envisioned a more independent, advocate body similar to the one proposed in earlier Campbell Report drafts.[26] Among those outraged at what had happened to the HEC, he soon found himself the governor's key adviser on health.

This role, though, had severe limits. As coordinator, he had few formal powers and a staff so small that he eventually had to rely on the IBHE for additional staff work. The IBHE proved to be firmly entrenched as the major political arena for budgetary wrangling and planning activities, since neither the governor nor the legislature wanted to get too deeply into the higher education political mire. This, then, is where the governor's coordinator would have to exert whatever influence he could muster.

Perhaps the most open conflict between Dr. Lepper and the University of Illinois developed over the question of whether the state should approve a new, 500-bed replacement teaching hospital the university had long sought. The detailed story of how the university ultimately prevailed is remarkably byzantine, and consequently it is beyond the scope of this study. Suffice it to say, the major objections can basically be summarized under these headings: (1) concern about over-bedding in the community; (2) the university had been so convincing about the advantages of using existing clinical facilities, why can't they do more of the same? and (3) concern over financing the $60 million project.[27]

Interestingly, during the debate over financing, it was pointed out that the $10 million annual deficit of the University of Illinois Hospital was subsidized by the higher education budget. The bulk of this deficit derives from the fact that 40 percent of the patients in the hospital are nonpaying persons without Medicare, Medicaid, or private insurance and also from the subsidization of the hospital's teaching program.[28]

Aside from the U. of I. hospital decision, a major concern beginning in 1974 for IBHE and the HEC was the task of producing Master Plan IV. This new plan would allow for an opportunity to assess past achievements and reexamine future goals—not only for health professions education but for all of higher education within the board's domain. Unlike previous efforts, the board would not establish blue-ribbon committees like the Campbell Commission. Rather, it would rely on what was described as "a blend whereby the existing agencies, boards, staffs, institutions and committees provide much of the technical input into the plan, tempered with the advice and recommendations of the public-at-large throughout the process." This was seen as the best way to satisfy the need to "recognize all who have a viewpoint," yet also involve "those who will have to implement the plan's recommendations."[29]

In terms of medical education support, the recommendations eventually evolving from the Master Plan IV enterprise reaffirmed previous commitments and goals first articulated in 1968—regionalization, aid to private schools, and expanding capacity through use of existing facilities. Although the Campbell Report acknowledged the important role of graduate medical education in overcoming geographic and specialty maldistribution, Master Plan IV contained generous provisions designed to assist medical schools in expanding their network of residency programs.

To this end, the schools and their affiliates would receive the following in state support: (a) one-time capital grant of $10,000 for each new appropriately approved first-year residency position in the primary-care specialties; and (b) an annual operating grant of $5,000 for each new first-year primary-care residency position and $2,500 for each new first-year nonprimary-care residency position. The medical schools—both public and private—receiving this money are expected to work toward having as many first-year residency positions as they have medical graduates. They also are to give priority to recruiting graduates of Illinois medical schools and to emphasize primary-care residencies, which are to make up one-half each school's total positions.[30]

The recommendations to continue growth in the medical education sector must be viewed in the context of the overall Master Plan IV report, which emphasized hard times ahead. A Chicago *Tribune* columnist reported: "The document has aroused scores of college and university administrators and faculty members because it stands not as an advocate for higher education but as a restraining force."[31] The educational community did not believe the board should be resigned to a fate of tighter financing from the state. Rather, it should more actively advocate a higher share of revenues for higher education instead of preaching increased productivity and reallocation of internal resources. Further, they were concerned over what was considered an invasion of their own proper jurisdictions—the size, type, and quality of programs offered. Teacher education was one particular battleground. But within the health field, one could see a turnabout in the perception of the nurse supply. The result was the following recommendation: "No new educational programs for practical nurses, associate degree nurses, diploma nurses, or baccalaureate degree nurses should be established unless a compelling need can be demonstrated.[32]

What does the future hold for physician training in Illinois? For the immediate future, the major issue will probably remain how steadily the medical schools can proceed toward increased enrollment goals and to what extent they can expand their network of graduate medical education. The public schools are concerned that unless incremental funds are made available to them they cannot expand their capacity and maintain quality.[33] So far, medical education has managed to remain the favored child of higher education. How long this will continue, however, depends on a number of factors.

Even with its particular status, medical education funding is ultimately tied to the fate of the higher education budget. For example, the delayed opening of the clinical program at the University of Illinois Urbana campus has been attributed directly to across-the-board cutbacks in the higher education budget—a situation that forced the university administrators to choose between medical education and other programs. Yet, unlike cutbacks in most other academic departments, the general community, which stood to gain from increased medical services, is more likely to make its feelings known to public officials. "Getting this program back into operation," read a Danville newspaper editorial, "will require considerable effort on the part of local citizens to convince all those on the State level that there is community support and need for such a program."[34]

The dynamic tension between "public" demand for more doctors and the limits imposed by the higher education budget has resulted in restrained growth (with the emphasis on "growth"). The question is what will happen if either public demand wanes or the higher education budget is squeezed. Enterprising medical schools under these circumstances will no doubt seek other means of maintaining their programs, either in the area of patient care of research. How successful they will prove to be depends upon future federal patient-care reimbursement practices and policies on overhead for externally funded research.

IMPLEMENTATION: ALTERNATIVES CONSIDERED

In the course of implementation, circumstances often arise that create pressure to deviate from or supplement the original plan. This section describes two instances in which such pressures developed and how Illinois officials responded.

A major concern expressed in the Campbell Report was that the additional resources applied to increasing the physician supply be used in a way that would redress the problems of service in shortage areas. Actually there had been a long-standing loan program sponsored by the Illinois State Medical Society and the Illinois Agricultural Association whereby potential medical school candidates from rural areas are screened and recommended for admission to the University of Illinois. Those who are granted admission (approximately 35 annually) receive a loan in exchange for an agreement to practice for a minimum period in certain rural areas of the state. Seventy participants in the program since 1948 have located their practices in rural areas after completing their service period.[35]

Several strategies were developed and employed under the direction of the Board of Higher Education in the hopes of further ameliorating the situation in shortage areas. One approach had involved the regionalization of medical education with new schools in Peoria, Rockford, and Springfield. Another approach revolved around the establishment of new primary-care residences. A belief that medical students who obtained their clinical training in community hospitals would be more likely to consider this as an alternative to suburban practice led to more medical school-community hospital affiliations. Finally, "aggressive recruitment programs" for minority students were instituted by the medical schools. From about 1970 to 1975, the minority enrollment in the state's medical schools was said to have increased from 3 to 10 percent; black enrollment increased from 1 to 6 percent.[36]

Despite this strong attack on distribution problems, the board encountered pressure from various groups who advocated alternative solutions. The first involved a forgiveness loan proposal from the General Assembly; the second involved political pressure to transform a dying inner-city hospital into a medical school affiliate.

The Forgiveness Loan Proposal

The predominant orientation of the board and its staff favored long-range programmatic efforts of the type described above. As illustrated in Table 5.5, physicians who received all of their training in Illinois are much more likely to remain than those who complete only part of their

Table 5.5. Retention of Physicians Trained in Illinois

Type of Training Obtained in Illinois	*Number of Physicians Practicing In Ill.*	*Elsewhere*	*Percent Retention*
Medical school			
a. Only	843	6,209	12
b. Plus intern *or* resident	3,256	4,523	42
c. Plus intern *and* resident	3,054	1,290	70
d. Subtotal: medical schools	7,153	12,022	37
Graduate medical education only			
a. Intern *or* resident	2,981	8,073	27
b. Intern *and* resident	2,002	3,473	37
c. Subtotal: graduate	4,983	11,546	30
Subtotal: Physicians training in Illinois	12,136	23,568	
No Training in Illinois	2,065		

Source: Illinois Board of Higher Education, "Tuition/Forgivable Loan Programs for Medical, Dental, and Veterinary Medicine Schools," 8 November 1974.

education—including internship and residency—within the state. This would seem to indicate the need for a comprehensive approach if the aim is to retain health professionals within the state.

Nonetheless, the possibility of a more dramatic payoff through some system of medical student loans with a service pay-back provision or direct financial incentives to practice in shortage areas was also considered. In November 1974, a report of Health Education Commission noted:

> The confluence of the high costs of the expansion of health professions education in Illinois and the perceived need to more directly address the problem of maldistribution of health manpower has spurred interest in the establishment of a mechanism whereby the student is required to bear a larger share of the educational cost (while, at the same time, ensuring that access to low-income groups is not reduced) and some further in-roads can be made with regard to geographical distribution.[37]

In considering the practicality of a forgivable loan program, the staff pointed out that there is little evidence to suggest how high tuition would need to be raised before the physician would be unlikely to buy out of his obligation. While some merit was recognized in seeking to achieve tuition parity among Illinois' state medical schools, as well as bringing it in line with the generally higher levels of tuition in out-of-state institutions, federal activity prompted a "wait-and-see" attitude. The rationale was expressed as follows:

> With the prospects being good for the establishment of a sizable Federal forgiveable loan, albeit the details are yet uncertain, caution should be exercised

in developing such a program in Illinois. The possible flow of Federal dollars into the State should not be jeopardized nor should Illinois unnecessarily duplicate a federal program. Rather, a complementary approach to the emerging Federal programs should be sought.[38]

Having reconfirmed its commitment to "long-run solutions," the board was faced with a resolution passed by the General Assembly requesting the formulation of a program for the admission of medical school applicants who agree to serve in areas of physician need in Illinois. After careful negotiation, the board and its staff convinced legislative leaders of the advisability of waiting in light of congressional activity and the board's own efforts to produce an updated master plan.[39]

The Provident Hospital Affair

In a Chicago *Sun-Times* article with the dramatic title, "Death Stalks a Hospital, Once-proud Provident Victim of a New Era," the executive director of the decaying South Side institution gave the newspaper an encapsulated history of the hospital—a history common to many ghetto hospitals across the country.

This hospital (founded in 1891) had been "the" hospital for black physicians. They graduated from schools like Howard and Meharry and came here for their residency. When they finished the highest level of training they usually resided in this area with staff privileges at Provident.[40]

When predominantly white hospitals in the 1960s began to admit blacks, Provident began to lose its private patients, who had helped defray the cost of treating indigent patients. Without the cash reserve to make repairs and purchase new equipment, the institution further declined, losing its internship program.

Having been informed by the state that it would have to close its doors by 1977 unless a replacement facility was built, the Provident board of directors began seeking funds not only to replace their 200 beds but to construct a 500-bed facility. Cook County Hospital, with more than 35 percent of its patients coming cross-city from Provident's service area, agreed to help insure the medical and financial viability of the new hospital by, among other ways, referring patients and providing medical staff to the new facility. The major problem was financing the $93 million project and finding a medical school willing to affiliate.

One of the prime sources of funds to build the hospital would have to be federal grants and loans. Yet HEW had its doubts about whether a 500-bed hospital was feasible. "Needs get confused with ability to pay," said one federal official. "We know there's a need there, but Provident could not carry this kind of debit requirement." As an alternative, HEW suggested a 340-bed hospital, projected at a cost of $58 million.[41]

In early 1976, Governor Walker sent a letter to the Chairman of the Board of Higher Education. In his communication, the governor pointed to the use of community hospitals in Springfield, Peoria, and Rockford to train physicians and suggested that "Provident Hospital's planned new physical facilities and intended expansion programs in both the inpatient and outpatient areas are such that they should easily become a key unit in the clinical educational programs.''[42]

In response to the governor's request to lay out the options for using South Side hospitals as health education sites, the Board of Higher Education staff prepared a report outlining the three major alternatives:

1. An affiliation with an existing medical school, like the University of Chicago, located near Provident Hospital, or the University of Illinois, which had gained experience in the use of community hospitals.

2. Establish a new medical school oriented toward enrolling minority students.

3. Affiliations with several medical schools that would help administer primary-care residencies and continuing education programs.[43]

All of these options entail a number of difficult questions yet to be resolved at the time the research for this book was completed. There remained questions of accreditation, the role of Cook County Hospital, and institutional responsibility for financing and operating residency programs. Unless enormous pressure was brought to bear, what medical school is likely to take on such a task voluntarily? Given the unsettling intrainstitutional effects of previous community hospital affiliations, along with the uncertainty inherent in the reimbursement picture, added to the particularly shaky state of Provident's finances, it would require an act of pure altruism on the part of a medical school to agree to affiliation.

No doubt the community could also make a strong case. After all, one major rationale for the massive state funding of medical education was to alleviate inner-city shortages. Would minority medical students trained in white medical schools be likely to practice in ghetto areas? A well-equipped hospital with educational programs situated in the inner city would surely improve the chances of attracting physicians while providing a source of care to the community.

CONCLUSION

Awareness of a social problem and willingness to combat it are obviously different. Early studies in Illinois indicate awareness of both physician out-migration and rural towns without doctors, yet not much corrective action was taken. Illinois mobilized only after the federal government took the first plunge. While the prospect of federal grant money was a factor, federal initiatives more likely served to focus public attention on the issue and convince state politicians that expanding the supply of physicians was an appropriate goal.

Once the state political machinery was mobilized, however, the leadership went further and faster than the federal government. Years of congressional deliberation had unearthed a good deal of information and had stimulated new ideas about medical education. The Campbell

Commission took these several strands, banked on the promise of federal support, and fashioned a plan for the State of Illinois. The Illinois Board of Higher Education and its Health Education Commission transformed an insightful analysis into an expanded and innovative medical education system. Meanwhile, the governor and General Assembly managed to provide a *relatively* stable source of funds to the plan. The plan itself has undergone constant revision.

Good social planning must be sensitive to political realities. The Campbell Commission did this well. However, the data gathered and the recommendations that followed must be tied together. Techniques for assessing manpower needs are primitive, yet one is forced to wonder whether the approach adopted was indeed the most efficient means of providing care to the ten percent of the population who, the commission's survey concluded, were without adequate medical services.

Modest inroads have been made in minority enrollment, retaining physicians in the state, and developing the capability of semirural areas to attract physicians and provide more health services. While enrollment increases have been achieved, the overwhelming demand for admission has not diminished the percentage of qualified residents who are unable to gain entrance.

Until the graduates of this period of expansion have settled into practice, it will be difficult to reach a final assessment of state-federal action. It seems unlikely, however, that any revolutionary changes in practice patterns are in the offing. Yet one legacy from these policies that bears careful scrutiny is the developing role of the academic medical center as, in the words of AAMC President John A. D. Copper, "convenient handles with which to manipulate the entire medical care system." How the academic medical center relates to the use of community health-care facilities as training sites for new physicians is the focus of the next chapter.

NOTES

1. Illinois, Board of Higher Education, *Education in the Health Fields for State of Illinois*, vols. I and II, June 1968.

2. Illinois, Board of Higher Education, "Summary of Expenditures of State-Appropriated Funds for Health Related Programs," 2 October 1975. Data also provided by Dr. James T. McGill, deputy director for Academic and Health Affairs, Illinois Board of Higher Education.

3. Pierre de Vise, "Physician Migration from Inland to Coastal States: Antipodal Examples of Illinois and California," *Journal of Medical Education* 48 (February 1974): 146–47.

4. *Report of the Commission to Survey Higher Education Facilities in Illinois*, January 1945, pp. 43–44.

5. Edward F. Potthoff, Trends in Medical Services and Training Facilities in Illinois (Urbana: Bureau of Institutional Research, University of Illinois, 1959), pp. 5, 9.

6. Gilbert Y. Steiner and Romayne R. Ponleithner, *Staff Report to the Committee to Recommend a State Plan for Public Education* (Springfield: Illinois Joint Council on Higher Education, 1961), pp. 176–77.

7. U.S., Department of Health, Education, and Welfare, *The Advancement of Medical Research and Education through the Department of Health, Education, and Welfare:*

Final Report of the Secretary's Consultants on Medical Research and Education, June 1958 (known as the Bayne-Jones report); and *Physicians for a Growing America: Report of the Surgeon General's Consultant Group on Medical Education, 1959* (known as the Bane Report).

8. Rosemary Stevens, *American Medicine and the Public Interest* (New Haven: Yale University Press, 1971), p. 365.

9. Robert H. Salisbury, "Report to Carnegie Commission on Higher Education," summarized in Heinz Eulau and Harold Quinley, *State Officials and Higher Education: A Survey of the Opinion and Expectations of Policy Makers in Nine States* (New York: McGraw-Hill, 1970), pp. 5–8.

10. Ibid., pp. 6–7.

11. Illinois, Board of Higher Education, *A Master Plan for Higher Education in Illinois*, July 1964, p. 44.

12. Illinois, 75th General Assembly, House Bill 1190 (1965).

13. Illinois, *Education in the Health Fields*, 1, p. vi.

14. Interview with Dr. Donald J. Casely, Vice Chancellor, University of Illinois at the Medical Center, Chicago.

15. Illinois, Board of Higher Education, Executive Director's Report no. 68, 10 September 1968.

16. Letter from George L. Clements, Chairman, Illinois Board of Higher Education to Emory Williams, Chairman, Health Education Commission, 13 June 1969.

17. "Minutes of the Illinois Board of Higher Education," 3 February 1970.

18. Letter from Governor Richard B. Ogilvie to Chairman, Illinois Board of Higher Education, 20 January 1970.

19. "Minutes of the Illinois Board of Higher Education," 3 February 1970.

20. Ibid.

21. Letter from George L. Clements, Chairman, Illinois Board of Higher Education to Harold H. Hines, Jr., 8 February 1972.

22. Letter from Commission members and telegram from Dr. Homer M. Kimmich, quoted in *The People's Health*, Comprehensive Health Planning, Inc., of Metropolitan Chicago, August 1972.

23. "Minutes of the Illinois Board of Higher Education," 7 January 1975.

24. "Minutes of the Illinois Board of Higher Education," 1 October 1974.

25. Ibid.

26. Interview with Dr. Mark Lepper, Director, State Comprehensive Health Planning Agency, 24 November 1975.

27. "Minutes of the Illinois Board of Higher Education," 7 May 1974.

28. Ibid.

29. "Minutes of the Illinois Board of Higher Education," 2 July 1974.

30. Illinois, Board of Higher Education, *A Master Plan for Post-secondary Education in Illinois*, March 1976, pp. 68–77.

31. Chicago *Tribune*, 12 November 1975.

32. Illinois, *Master Plan*, March 1976, p. 69.

33. University of Illinois, "Comments on IBHE Draft of a Master Plan for Postsecondary Education in Illinois," November 1975.

34. *Commercial News*, Danville, Illinois, 23 January 1976.

35. Ellen Sax, *Incentive Programs: Promoting Practice in Underserved Areas* (New York: National Health Council, 1976) pp. 2–3.

36. "Minutes of the Illinois Board of Higher Education," 4 March 1975.

37. Illinois, Board of Higher Education, Health Education Commission, "Tuition/Forgivable Loan Programs for Medical, Dental, and Veterinary MEdicine Schools," 8 November 1974.

38. Ibid.

39. Interview with James T. McGill.

40. Chicago *Sun-Times* 5 September 1976.

41. ibid.

42. Letter from Governor Daniel Walker to Dr. Donald Prince, Chairman, Illinois Board of Higher Education, 27 January 1976.

43. Illinois, Board of Higher Education, "Background Paper on Potential Use of South Side Chicago Hospitals as Affiliates for Health Professions Education Programs," n.d., pp. 16–18.

6

Institutional and Community Politics

As the medical schools left the confines of their traditional walls, they had to learn to deal with community hospitals, local politicians, and local practitioners. They had helped to create a new world inhabited by satellite clinics, area health education centers, preceptorships, continuing education, and minority recruitment programs; now they had to learn to live in that new world.

THE UNIVERSITY OF ILLINOIS

In one respect, the Campbell Report was probably the key force to push the University of Illinois toward expansion. However, internal activity and interest within the university itself were responsible for priming the institution to act quickly and decisively when the opportunity became available.

A much discussed 1964 report by Dr. Lester J. Evans on education for the health professions,[1] calling for university leadership in meeting the health needs of the state, came at a time when the university feared its mission as a "comprehensive state university" was being threatened by suggestions that its growth be limited in favor of new institutions.[2] Thus the Evans report, while tapping the popular belief that university *medical* centers should become comprehensive *health* centers by integrating the resources of the whole institution, also provided a rationale for seeking to maintain the university's preeminence within the state.

Construction of new facilities for the university's colleges of Medicine, Nursing, and Pharmacy was under way by 1965 with the assistance of the federal government. The effect of federal requirements for large local matching funds was noted by the university's President, David D. Henry, when he pointed out: "[This puts] a serious strain on the effort to distribute available funds equitably throughout the University for continuing operation as well as for new facilities and new enterprises."[3] Presumably, the strain would be even greater if new medical schools were to compete for limited state matching funds.

The activities of an office of research in medical education—which for years had studied admissions policy, career patterns of graduates, and quality of instruction—along with the efforts of a special faculty committee, produced the following recommendations, calling for the College of Medicine to:

1. Increase substantially its production of physicians.
2. Assume leadership in investigating, with other colleges of the university, various approaches to greater efficiency and productivity in the basic education of personnel for the health professions and explore the need for further basic science facilities.
3. Assume leadership in investigating the possibility of establishing additional affiliations in order to provide the clinical facilities necessary for expansion.[4]

By the time the Campbell Report was in preparation, the university had a framework within which to operationalize its broad policy declaration, and subsequently it had a mandate to implement recommendations as well as the public money to support the implementation.

The doubling of student capacity at the University of Illinois was not accomplished simply by expanding the facilities at the Chicago medical center campus, but by reorganizing the college into a regional system of six semi-autonomous components (five schools and a group of Chicago community hospitals). The two basic science schools have responsibility for the concentrated first year of nonclinical course work. The three clinical schools in Chicago, Peoria (180 miles southwest of Chicago), Rockford (100 miles west of Chicago), and their respective affiliated hospitals then take over for the remainder of the student's medical education. The sixth school is composed of the allied health programs.

Sensitive to the political ramifications of regionalizing a major public medical school in this fashion, university officials hoped to minimize local community conflict that could arise from injudicious behavior by the university in its enthusiasm to expand.

Each city had three vigorous and interested general hospitals and negotiating affiliation agreements with each might have seemed a reasonable way to begin. After lengthy deliberation the alternate path of community planning and decision-making was adopted in order to insure an integrated health professions education and health service delivery system, and to avoid placing the University in the middle of any potential struggles among institutions vying for status and power. Recognizing the merits of such a view both Peoria and Rockford created Health Education Foundations, organizations that included physicians, hospital administrators, hospital trustees, and community leaders, to work with University representatives in developing guiding principles for institutional interrelationships and preliminary organizational plans.[5]

Traditionally, University of Illinois medical students received most of their clinical training in the three hospitals located in the vicinity of the West Side campus. With the addition of the six hospitals making up the metropolitan hospital group, the resources of the university were considerably extended. However, questions of governance, budget, appointments, and promotion have not easily been resolved. For instance, discussions of whether to have one or two clinical schools within Chicago have not been readily resolved.[6]

Figure 6.1 illustrates the complexity of university organization. While the College of Medicine's policy is to delegate authority for educational program operation to the deans and directors of the individual schools, decisions on program coordination and resource allocation are reserved for the executive dean, who chairs an Administrative Advisory Council made up of the heads of the component schools. An academic council, composed of deans and elected faculty members, has final authority over academic policies and programs involving such matters as admissions, faculty promotion, and appraisal of student progress.

As one would expect, expansion and administrative reorganization have not proceeded without tension, suspicions, and disgruntlement. From the beginning, elements within the faculty were concerned that the quality of graduates would decline as students took their training in distant communities, and that the research enterprise would suffer as emphasis was placed on the production of family doctors. A good deal of anxiety was expressed over issues of tenure and promotions as it became clear that the standard criteria relying on research output might not be applicable for the new types of faculty being recruited.[7]

As the anxieties and problems of the past dissipate—or to be more cynical, go underground—the university, looking to the future, has begun to work on a new set of objectives. The next steps for the University of Illinois will be a necessary consequence of earlier ones. The years of expansion must be followed by a reassessment of institutional commitments and administrative control. A major part of this reassessment will undoubtedly involve the governance of its outposts in Rockford and Peoria, as well as the continued management of its Area Health Education System.

ROCKFORD SCHOOL OF MEDICINE

The following statement, excerpted from a document designed to convey the "concept" of the Rockford School of Medicine, provides a

Figure 6.1 University of Illinois at the Medical Center

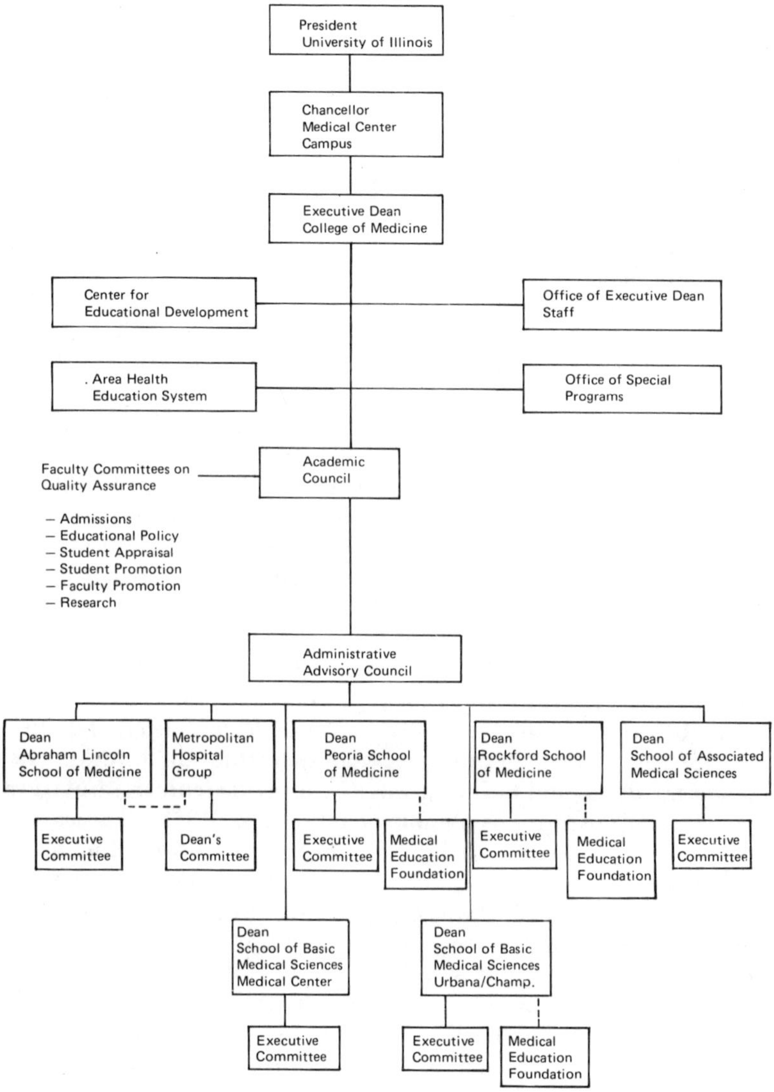

Source: George C. Miller, *State of the College*. University of Illinois, College of Medicine, January 1974.

useful springboard for the discussion of the institution as a political entity.

> It is planned that the RSM be seen by Rockford's citizens as a community institution, operated with the expertise and capability of the University of Illinois, rather than RSM being identified purely as a unit of University which happens to be located in Rockford.[8]

Given the traditional predilection of medical schools to view themselves as national (or at least state) resources, what are the political implications of a medical school that considers itself a "community institution"—one in fact that is administratively tied to a parent in a distant city? While the Chicago medical campus, like most older urban medical centers, has had to come to terms with its immediate community, it does not consider itself a "community institution." Newer medical schools, however, and especially those removed from large urban settings, often owe their existence to the persistence of local community leaders who marshaled the needed political and economic resources. The question is, does the community play a continuing role in the development and policies of the school it has helped to establish?

The focal point of activity to bring a medical school to Rockford was at first the Community Hospital Council, a group of civic and medical leaders who saw the potential of the Campbell Commission. After publication of the Campbell Report, which recommended Rockford as the site for a University of Illinois satellite, the Hospital Council organized the Rockford Medical Education Foundation to work with the university on site selection, the search for a dean, hospital affiliations, and the recruitment of local physicians to serve on the faculty.[9]

Dr. Robert L. Evans began his tenure as dean in 1971, and one year later the first class of 20 students began their training at RSM. The site chosen for the school building was a former tuberculosis sanitarium. A formal relationship was established between RSM and health-care facilities in the city, which includes three hospitals (totaling approximately 1,100 acute beds) and a mental health center serving nine counties. Also established was a community health center program, four ambulatory-care facilities in the surrounding towns of Belvidere, Durand, Mount Morris, and Kirkland.

This program was adopted after rejecting two other models of providing students with clinical experience in ambulatory care. The model of a multispecialty outpatient clinic serving mainly charity patients was seen by the curriculum planners as a "brown bench clinic pattern" that "teach[es] a form of medicine shorn of human empathy." Alternatively, the use of the private offices of the faculty was perceived to be useful only in selected instances because of a number of drawbacks, including lack of qualified individuals who could provide the space and time required for fitting a student into an office routine, not to mention the loss of an estimated 30 to 50 percent of the physician's income, which the school would be obliged to replace.

The community health center program was finally settled upon as the most satisfactory means of providing appropriate clinical experience to the students as well as more care to underserved communities. The program, which the school proudly proclaims to be "the first effort of its kind in the United States," involves a center staffed by two or more full-time primary-care physicians serving as role models for the students and providing continuing personal care for a patient population. Approximately 25 percent of the student's time at Rockford is spent at these centers, which strive to use up-to-date techniques in organizing a practice (e.g., problem-oriented records), as well as integrative professional review of quality of care into the center's activities. The centers are expected to maintain operation through fee-for-service charges to patients, since the university only pays for the salaries of the teacher-physicians. (The Kirkland center proved unable to attract a sufficient clientele and as a result had to discontinue operations.) As the size of the school increases, the number of centers are also expected to increase.[10]

Following the tenets of the Campbell Report, Rockford's dean, Robert Evans, enthusiastically embraced the goals of effective medical education and service to the community:

> We will educate a doctor at one-tenth of the capital cost of traditional medical schools and two-fifths of operating cost. This cost savings will be achieved by local physicians giving time as teachers and by utilizing hospital facilities. We won't have the expense of building a 1,000 bed university hospital and a series of clinics that require large numbers of people to man them. Rockford is getting a tremendous bargain and so is the state.[11]

In practice, however, the task of mobilizing preexisting local resources is not always easy, and it sometimes places the medical school in an uncomfortable position in the local political structure. One instance of this can be seen in attempts to expand the school's Belvidere health center.

Over the years it became clear to many in the community that the two hospitals in Belvidere were seriously underused and that duplication of facilities was costly. Yet, several attempts to merge the two hospitals had failed. Meanwhile, the Rockford School of Medicine was hoping that the two hospitals would agree to house clinic offices for the health center program. Instead, one of the hospitals offered land to build a clinic. Dean Evans responded to the offer as follows: "We are declining [St. Joseph's offer of land] in order that it be clearly understood that the Rockford School of Medicine does not wish to promulgate divisiveness or prolong competition in the hospital care delivery system for Belvidere."[12] The mayor of Belvidere, however, wanted to know why the School of Medicine was buying land and installing expensive equipment that the two hospitals already possessed. "The money that is being spent is our tax dollars," wrote Mayor Whalen in the local newspapers. "It would not have to be spent if the hospitals would consolidate, but at the present time, the Rockford School of Medicine is not getting into a community problem."[13] Dean Evans responded by acknowledging that the hospital situation was indeed a drain on resources, but that the operation of the health center was not supported by state taxes but patient fees.[14]

Even retrospectively it is not altogether clear whether the school should have entered into this local political squabble. The costs of alienating segments of the community may not have been worth the risks to a fledgling institution. However, the fact that state taxes were not directly supporting the health-care center is no excuse for an institution predicated on the principle of effective use of resources to contributing to a further duplication. There are, of course, no easy answers. In the end, the university got its new health center primarily through private philanthropy.[15]

Despite the inevitable periodic friction between the medical school and its environment, a sense of proprietary interest has naturally developed within the community for the institution. This was clearly demonstrated in the instance of Dean Evan's ouster by the Executive Dean of the University of Illinois School of Medicine, Dr. William Grove. The immediate reasons for the precipitous dismissal were reported in the local press as one of "irreconcilable differences" between Grove and Evans.[16] It is generally believed that from central administration's viewpoint, Evans was seen as undermining central authority by refusing to acquiesce to university statutes and procedures.

Aside from the relationship of personalities contributing to the incident, it is worthwhile viewing the dismissal for its structural implications. *The New Physician*, a national publication interested in the Rockford situation, interviewed faculty and students concerning the firing of Evans and described their views about the problems of "semiautonomy" in a decentralized medical school system.

> The way the students and faculty see it, the root of the problem lies in the lack of clear division of authority between the University and the school. . . . They see Grove's firing of Evans as a sign of things to come. . . . The University had said that its goal was decentralizing medical education in Illinois. The people at Rockford suspect that the University really has in mind expansion—and there's a big difference between the two.[17]

In addition to the intrauniversity aspects of the affair, the community also began to express its displeasure at the firing of the popular Evans. For example, State Representative W. Timothy Simms, a Republican from Rockford, directed the threat of a formal legislative inquiry in a letter to Dr. John Corbally, University of Illinois president. The letter posed the possibility of an examination of "the operation of the school of medicine, both at Rockford and Chicago, and into the ability of your administration to continue its function of directing the University of Illinois." Rep. Simms went on to say: "The philosophy, curriculum and the leadership of the Rockford School of Medicine have attained national recognition and total acceptance by the Rockford community under the direction of Robert Evans."[18]

No doubt, top university officials and Grove himself were taken aback by the publicity and furor over what they presumed to be strictly an internal problem. Perhaps the incident may never have occurred if different personalities were involved or if it had been handled more diplomatically. Nonetheless, it may also be indicative of the more general phenomenon of organizational expansion. As medical schools are pressured to reach out geographically and as decision-making becomes a corporate responsibility, medical school leadership is likely to encounter administrative problems they have never before faced.

PEORIA SCHOOL OF MEDICINE

Like its sister satellite in Rockford, the Peoria School of Medicine was brought into being with the aid of local community leaders who also perceived the institution as part of an ongoing civic effort to develop the community. The great test of organizational survival for the Peoria school, however, came at the beginning in a struggle over site selection—a struggle that well illustrates the complex interaction of the various levels of government. So complex were the interactions that local notables themselves marveled at the eventual resolution of the problem, or at what one official called the "synergy of three, maybe four, levels of government . . . federal, state, local and the University of Illinois." Adding his comments on the occasion of the ground-breaking ceremony, U.S. Rep. Robert H. Michel (R. 18th), remarked: "I would like to think of the beginning of this project as a real prime example of the 'new federalism.' It really takes some extraordinary people locally and statewide to implement these [federal] programs."[19]

The original conception of a medical school in Peoria dates back more than ten years prior to the entrance of a first class of students in 1972. It was at this time that the Peoria Medical Society established the Medical School Exploratory Committee to investigate the possibility of an institution, such as nearby Bradley University, taking on the task. The committee eventually came to the conclusion that financial support would not be easy to come by. However, in 1965, they managed to convince State Rep. Ronald Hurst of Peoria to sponsor the bill in the Illinois legislature, and this ultimately led to the establishment of the Campbell Commission.[20]

The next step was the organization of a community-wide committee, which elected as its head the chairman of the board of the Caterpillar Tractor Company. This committee, known as the Peoria Medical Society Advisory Committee, included representatives of the local hospitals, the medical society, and the Association of Commerce. Thus when the Campbell Commission was ready to hold hearings, the advisory committee was ready to testify and present a strong case. Once the decision was made to use Peoria as one of the decentralized schools of the University of Illinois, the committee created the Peoria Board for Medical Education, Inc. with little delay, establishing numerous subcommittees and task forces to work with the university.

The Peoria Medical School began its operations by leasing space from

Bradley University while negotiations over a final site were taking place. This was one of the major problems facing Dr. Nicholas J. Cotsonas, Jr., the newly appointed dean. The delicacy of the situation is suggested by Dean Cotsonas's own words:

> Because the Peoria School of Medicine is a regional semiautonomous school within the College of Medicine of the University of Illinois, Deputy Executive Dean Richard M. Magraw of the College of Medicine and I suggested to the University Administration the desirability of seeking input from the community. After considerable discussion, I approached the Peoria Board for Medical Education, Inc., and reviewed with the board not only the desirability for such input but emphasized what a significant departure this was for the University of Illinois. I asked the board to appoint a small committee to this confidential assignment.[21]

The university along with a consulting firm concluded that the best site was a suburban one located north of Parkview Cemetery. The Parkview site, as it became known, appealed to University officials because of its neutral location in relation to the major existing health facilities, the relatively low cost of the land, and its potential for future expansion.[22]

The professional community, however, vehemently opposed this site and favored a more centrally located area, one near the St. Francis and Methodist hospitals. The Peoria Medical Society passed a resolution strongly recommending this site. Even the provisional faculty of the School of Medicine voted to endorse the medical society's resolution in a meeting at which one participant commented: "But what it seems to me and also to others is that it doesn't matter a damn about where we want our school—the site's already been chosen." Others reacted negatively to remarks Dean Grove had made during a newspaper interview, in which he was quoted: "If the Peoria School of Medicine is closely associated with the hospitals, it will be continuing in the old way." Grove explained: "The medical education field has been concerned with the treatment and diagnosis of disease since 1910. The future is in the detection and prevention of disease and the promotion of health, all of which is done outside of hospitals." Apparently affronted by this comment, one doctor complained: "I don't think he [Dr. Grove] is being fair in his evaluation of Peoria doctors as being disease oriented and parochial because we want a particular site."[23]

To complicate matters further, the resourceful mayor of Peoria, Richard Carver, recognized that the downtown location of the medical school could provide him with the necessary leverage to get the federal urban-renewal funds he had been seeking. At that time, in late 1973, urban-renewal money that had been frozen under a Nixon Administration moratorium could be released only in exceptional circumstances. Officials from the Federal Department of Housing and Urban Development informed the mayor that if the medical school site could be changed to the downtown renewal area, the city would qualify for $7 million in emergency funding.[24]

Mayor Carver, anticipating the university's reluctance to reverse their minds on the Parkview site, decided to take his case before the Capital Development Board, a state agency responsible for recommending the release of state funds for medical school construction. Although the board had already approved the Parkview site, they decided to freeze these funds until a mediated settlement between the city and the board could be reached.

University officials entered negotiations determined to maintain their position. "No other group can adopt a site (for the Peoria School of Medicine) and tell us that's what we're going to do,"[25] said Chancellor Joseph Beagando of the university's medical center. Yet, pressures created by the prospect of federal millions could not be overcome by university administrators and trustees, who eventually agreed to the site change but not without a number of assurances from the city concerning barriers that might interfere with the construction timetable. This matter of a timetable was of particular concern to the medical school administrators, who had developed a certain amount of skepticism about the federal government. Said Dean Grove: "I've dealt long enough with the federal government to know you don't believe it until you see the check in your hand."[26]

In praise of the university's reversal, Mayor Carver proclaimed: "They have taken the initiative to support not only this community's medical needs but its redevelopment needs as well. The city will back them right down the line with all the technical support we can."[37]

What the Peoria and Rockford experience seems to exemplify is a more intricate picture of medical school expansion and intergovernmental relations than had been portrayed previously. The reasons for and the implementation of expansion involve more than just a determination of health manpower needs and the establishment of training programs; they also involve many overlapping concerns that cut across jurisdictional lines of decision-making.

AREA HEALTH EDUCATION SYSTEM

Having already established a regional framework, the University of Illinois was in a good position to compete for one of eleven Area Health Education Center (AHEC) contracts awarded by the federal government under provisions of the Comprehensive Health Manpower Training Act of 1971. The federal AHEC concept and Illinois' role in realizing it was neatly summed up by the university's executive medical dean:

> We have established medical schools outside Chicago using state funds. Now, with federal money, we will establish family practice residencies for graduate physicians, and we will educate nurses and various allied health professionals.
>
> The frequent pleas and advertisements by towns without doctors all over Illinois point up the necessity of AHEC's. But we are responding, as well, to the fact that a physician today needs an array of other health professions at his side if he is to be effective.[28]

In effect, the approach was to be the often-stated admonition, "You can't just parachute young doctors into rural areas without backing them up with support personnel and colleague interaction." The implication is that drastic measures aimed at enticing or coercing physicians into rural areas have only limited and short-term benefits. What is required is a long-range, rural development strategy.

After three years of a five-year contract, the Illinois AHEC program spent $3,727,542. Out of this sum, $501,048 was allotted to graduate medical education. Family practice residency programs were established in the four regions comprising the area health education system; and the first small group of residents to complete the programs appears to be accepting positions in the region where they trained. Other AHEC activities—health-team projects, continuing education, health-care-delivery research projects, and coordinating activities—impact more or less directly on the training of medical students as well.[29]

Despite the apparent advantages of federal funds to help move the university toward its regionalization goal, involvement with the federal government was not without problems. Those responsible at the university for operating the AHEC program identified several concerns in their annual reports. Perhaps the best two words to describe the nature of these concerns are "indefinite" and "inconsistent." They reported that "Many communities question the stability and intent of the federally funded AHEC program which advocates increased utilization of clinical institutions for education at a time marked by recent withdrawal of Federal funding for clinical medical education."[30]

This general lack of confidence in a stable federal policy had its roots in the extended uncertainty surrounding the impact of pending health planning and health manpower legislation. That contracts were written "without community input or approval by regulatory agencies within the State" no doubt also contributed to the level of skepticism. Added to this were the difficulties associated with HEW decentralization, which Illinois AHEC administrators claimed had created "problems in management and communications with regard to Federal and regional information needs and interpretation of the original contract." There has also been uneasiness over the direction federal evaluation of the AHEC project was taking in Illinois.[31]

In accepting the AHEC contract, the university had the job of taking the Carnegie Commission's ideal model of an Academic Health Science Center, related to another ideal model, called an Area Health Education Center, and adapting it to the realities of its own circumstances. In attempting to live up to the ideal—in other words, to fulfill the terms of the contract—the Illinois AHEC had to operate "*ahead* of existing policies and procedures of the University of Illinois," all of which tends to create pressures on existing administrative relationships. One sensitive area, for example, was the administration of funds for educational programs in nursing and allied health by the College of Medicine.[32]

The key concepts of health education reform—"interdisciplinary," "interinstitutional," and "regional"—are not easily operationalized by organizational structures designed in an earlier day. The accommodations require a greater concentration of power in a centralized authority.

Yet, no longer is this merely a dean with a small staff; it is the institutionalized deanship, a conglomerate of various coordinating, data-gathering, and policy-making units surrounding a university official. Pressure to relocate the AHEC contract administration from the College of Medicine to the chancellor's office is part of this trend.

SOUTHERN ILLINOIS UNIVERSITY

In the fall of 1973, a first-year class began its studies in a major new medical school built to serve the needs of southern and central Illinois, an underdeveloped, predominantly rural area of the state characterized by all the problems one would expect to find with the declining industries of mining and agriculture. Among those problems was a perceived physician shortage. The extent of this problem was elaborated in a 1964 study emanating from Southern Illinois University.

> The thirty-one Southern Illinois counties had a total of 731 registered physicians to serve a population of 1,054,996. Of the registered physicians, 31 were retired or not in active practice and an additional 104 were over 70 years of age. Seven hundred physicians in active practice to serve a population of 1,054,996 resulted in an average of 1,507 persons for each physician. This has been defined as a crisis situation in which the public health of the area might be jeopardized. When a more adequate standard of 742 persons per physician was applied, a need for 1,422 physicians was indicated. This meant that the number of physicians in Southern Illinois needed to be doubled if adequate service were to be made available to the people of the area.[33]

It was evident that any plans for expansion by the state of its medical school capacity would have to take into account the above statistics, the high concentration of medical schools in the Chicago area, and the political power of the downstate legislators. It was also evident that the aggressively expanding Southern Illinois University, a state institution that saw itself as a regional resource for economic development, would be the repository of a new medical school. The major question to resolve was how to find the appropriate community for the clinical part of the program.

Writing in the mid-1950s, Michael Davis, an early exponent of health-care reform, commented on "the rural medical problem"—a problem that he considered to be secondarily one of poverty.

> It is primarily one of education and organization. Its solution depends more on what rural people and their organization leaders understand, want, and will work for, than upon the views of county and state medical societies and the A.M.A. The cities and their suburbs have, as a rule, relatively sufficient medical personnel and facilities, so that their chief problem is to organize and finance available resources, whereas rural areas face the additional problems of obtaining more personnel and new capital funds.[34]

The potential sources of leadership Davis surmised were hospital trustees and medical educators; and indeed these two groups were instrumental in successfully promoting the state capitol, Springfield, as a site for the SIU medical school. An unsuspected source of leadership, however, came from the Sangamon County Medical Society.

The constrictionist policies of national and local organized medicine of which Davis was familiar had given way in the 1960s to an advocacy on behalf of increasing the physician supply, a change culminating in the joint AMA-AAMC policy statement of 1968.[35] One major reason for shifting attitudes was the passage of Medicare and Medicaid. These federal programs extended the trend of more stable medical-care financing—a trend that contributed greatly toward convincing rural physicians that they need not fear the competition and low incomes that prevailed during the Depression. These doctors, no doubt, also saw benefits that would accrue from a medical education program in the local hospitals. Interns and residents could perform housestaff services, and more specialists could be attracted into the area, permitting the patients of local GPs to be treated locally rather than in St. Louis or Chicago. Of course these benefits also could be accompanied by some negative consequences, not the least of which was potentially being professionally embarrassed by the presence of sophisticated medical educators and specialists.

Nonetheless, the local medical society lent its support—although perhaps somewhat guarded support—to the effort of attracting a medical school to Springfield. The boards of directors of the two major hospitals (St. John's and Memorial), like all hospital trustees, had visions of enhancing the prestige and size of their medical centers. And thus the Springfield Committee for Medical Education was born in July 1966, in time to prepare for December hearings of the Campbell Commission. The Springfield group later organized a two-day seminar in which they invited national experts "to share their experience with them and to spell out both the advantages and drawbacks of starting a major educational program in the health fields."[36] One doubts that anything these experts had to say about drawbacks would have dissuaded the committee from their objective of bringing medical education to Springfield. Yet, such conferences serve the purpose of providing publicity, rallying local public support, improving communication among decision-makers in a modest way, and sometimes even generating constructive ideas.

Shortly after the Campbell Commission published its report, the SIU trustees formally approved establishing a medical school in Springfield (April 1969), purchased land in the city (November 1970), signed affiliation agreements with the two Springfield hospitals (December 1970), and finally broke ground for Phase I of the construction program (December 1971).

If there is a raison d'etre for Southern Illinois University School of Medicine, it is to improve the health care of the citizens who live within its regions. This was the stated intention of the Campbell Commission, and this mission has been interpreted by the school:

> This has not been taken to mean that the school should provide health services directly to large segments of the population; it does reflect the school's

responsibility to direct its publicity funded resources in ways which advocate health in its broadest sense and to support the work of health professionals, institutions, citizens groups and state agencies engaged in developing approaches to assuring access by all citizens to acceptable, affordable and appropriate personal medical care.[37]

How has SIU operationalized this philosophy in structuring its program?

First, there is the admissions process. Over the years, researchers have attempted to discover key variables that would permit medical school admissions committees to select students likely to pursue specific kinds of careers in medicine. To date, there has been little success in predicting which applicants are most likely to practice primary care in a rural setting.

Nonetheless, SIU and state medical schools like it operate on the assumption that background characteristics of students are an aid to selecting students to fulfill the school's mission. As in the case of most medical schools today, there is no dearth of well-qualified applicants seeking to be admitted to SIU's program. For the 60 openings in 1974, there were 1,207 applicants. Those students who are "numerically qualified" (i.e., medical college admission test scores and grade-point average) are then subjected to three personal interviews to determine whether their personal qualities indicate a likelihood of remaining in Illinois and "potential physicianhood." The school admits only Illinois residents as undergraduates and claims that their approach to admissions "has resulted in the denial of candidates whose numerical indicators gave assurance of professional success as a provider of personal health care." Whether or not the school is completely successful in retaining its graduates in Illinois, it also sees its mission in part as increasing opportunities for Illinois residents to receive a medical education.[38]

In addition to its attempts to improve the admission process, SIU has also maintained with the help of federal funds a special recruitment and preparation program for racial minority students, women, veterans, and rural students from low-income families. In 1974, the Medical Education Preparatory Program (MED PREP) had a full-time recruiter and a faculty of six to teach tutorials in courses preparatory to medical education. The nondegree, open-ended program has ambitious goals: It is anticipated that eventually 70 to 80 percent of the graduates from the program will be accepted to SIU School of Medicine or to other medical schools.[39]

SIU medical school's outreach to the communities of southern and central Illinois entails several interrelated efforts. Aside from the undergraduate students its trains, the medical school also hopes to attract and retain residents. "Residency programs under development," so the school contends, "are based primarily upon the physician manpower needs of Central and Southern Illinois but reflect also the need of the school for balanced educational programs and the interests of affiliated hospitals in staffing for areas of specialty service and patient care."[40]

In other times and other places, these separate interests have not necessarily complemented one another. Yet SIU, by putting a premium on developing family practice programs, as well as involving area physicians in either part-time paid or volunteer teaching, hopes to create a kind of synergism in which the continuing education needs of practicing physicians and the health-care needs of the population are served by the school's pursuing its teaching mission. The establishment of regional health education centers—satellite continuing-education programs for practicing physicians and other health personnel in key areas around the region—is one device the school employs in its attempt to institutionalize having one's cake and eating it too. The stated purpose of these centers is "to enhance the regionalization and localization of health education and to assess the educational needs and desires of health care professionals within a specific geographic area."[41] The "meaningful relationships" and "partnership" that the school anticipates will develop with community physicians are also expected to lead to the development of residency training programs.

PRIVATE MEDICAL SCHOOLS

The notion of public support for private medical schools is consistent with a general concern within the higher education community over how to preserve diversity in light of the growing hegemony of public postsecondary education. One argument put forth in favor of governmental aid to the private sector is that public institutions would be required to take over at greater expense the tasks that private schools now perform. A more noble argument that some prefer, however, is one that stresses the private sector's contribution toward providing "certain major goods to innovation and differentiation."[42]

Illinois and other states had come to accept these arguments, and they are reflected in the Campbell Report. However, state aid to nonpublic institutions was to be carefully controlled and monitored, with accountability to the Board of Higher Education. This meant that funds would be appropriated to the board, which had the responsibility to determine the amounts to be requested from the General Assembly and then arrive at specific allocations for each institution. While the board would rely on a formula to determine allocations, the formula could be revised on the basis of the financial data on construction and operation costs that each participating school was required to submit.[43]

Even with the state subsidization plan, there was still some concern that Illinois private schools might succumb to financial pressures. Therefore the commission acknowledged the possibility of private schools entering the public system. Three modes of entry were suggested:

1. Direct entry through establishment of a relationship with a single state university offering a medical curriculum on the basis of a schools-within-a-college concept;
2. Entry through the establishment of a relationship with a single state

university not having a medical school or full medical curriculum at that time;

3. Entry through the establishment of a relationship with a consortium of state universities or colleges through the appropriate governance boards.[44]

The private schools of Illinois did not find it necessary to take these roads to financial solvency. Indeed, Rush Medical School, a private institution, was begun in the period after the commission completed its work. Also, the federal government disbursed more than $5 million in special-project funds for financial need to private schools.[45]

Like Mount Sinai Hospital in New York, Rush's Presbyterian-St Luke's Hospital saw limits to growth in the future and even eventual loss of prestige without its own medical school.[46] Chicago's well-known Michael Reese medical center, in the midst of the inner city, has been concerned about just this problem. The medical center's president had said: "It is clear that the center has the academic potential to be a major medical teaching center, and our affiliation with the University of Chicago does not fulfill that potential."[47] The University of Chicago with its own hospital is reluctant to develop a major teaching program at Michael Reese. Yet without a strong affiliation, the hospital often finds itself in a less competitive position for large research and project grants.

The problems associated with the financial viability of urban hospitals are enormously complex, and the complexity often merges with the tangled web of medical education. However, the more the physician supply is seen as being adequate and as the cost of medical school development escalates, it is difficult to see how nonpublic hospitals will be able to save themselves by starting their own medical schools.

Another variation on the theme of the private medical school-nonpublic hospital-public interest triangle can be seen in the attempts of Chicago Medical School to extricate itself from its inner-city location. When the school announced its plan to move to Downey, Illinois, forty miles from Chicago, the staff and board of its affiliate, Mount Sinai Hospital, threatened to break its ties with the school. As negotiations proceeded, the press took note. Eight department chairmen, arguing that the move would weaken Mt. Sinai's teaching programs, refused to move their offices and resigned from the school's faculty. Governor Walker deplored the move, saying that "The medical facilities are an integral part of the West Side and the services provided are essential to that area." He also pointed out that state funds were being spent to help the school.[48]

Nonetheless, Chicago Medical School did move its facilities to Downey, where it affiliated with the V.A. hospital and the Great Lakes Naval Hospital. The Mt. Sinai affiliation was picked up by Rush Medical School. Perhaps both the medical schools and the hospitals are better off, and maybe that is in the public interest. At any rate, neither the federal nor the state government chose to use the leverage of financial support to keep the school within the city.

Former IBHE staff member James T. McGill has estimated that the "long-run cost of adding an additional physician to the practice of medicine in Illinois, via the state program, is about $50,000." The total cost to the state for the program of aid to the five private medical schools approached $45 million by 1976, with $19 million of that sum devoted to construction support. McGill has also estimated the effect of the state expansion plan over and above the requirements imposed by the federal capitation program. His estimates can be seen in Table 6.1.[49]

Table 6.1. Comparative Enrollments in Five Private Illinois Medical Schools

Cumulative first-year enrollments: 1969-70 to 1975-76	*Absence of State Plan (estimated)*	*Illinois State Plan (actual)*	*Difference*
Illinois residents	1,235	2,067	832
Non-Illinois residents	1,776	1,717	–59
Total	3,011	3,784	773

The wisdom of this type of expenditure has been questioned by one economist who looked at the Illinois experience. Applying Donald Yett's and Frank Sloan's techniques for analyzing factors affecting medical school graduate migration patterns, James A. Dei Rossi concluded that "emphasis on medical school enrollment rather than internships and residency, is likely to be largely ineffectual in achieving the program goal of increasing future retention of graduates." The inference is that minimal benefits to the state would accrue from supporting undergraduate medical education in the private sector.[50]

The board and its staff, however, are apparently pleased with the performance of the private schools and have recommended in Master Plan IV annual operating grants of $4,200 per Illinois resident enrolled in these schools. In addition, the private medical schools have been encouraged to participate in the development of graduate medical education in community hospitals, for which, as has been discussed, generous public support is made available.[51]

THE FEDERAL GOVERNMENT AND ILLINOIS

As we have seen, federal influence on a state can operate in subtle ways. The availability of small sums of money from federally inspired programs like Comprehensive Health Planning and the Regional Medical program to help support state planning efforts is only one manifestation of the federal presence. Another less concrete manifestation is the effect of impending federal action on state-level policymakers: The decision to defer action on a state scholarship-forgiveness program is one case in point. Even more difficult to measure is the federal contribution toward creating a sense of public urgency about a problem such as the physician shortage. There is no way to judge to what extent Illinois and other states would have invested in medical education without the expectation of an eventual federal role, without the stream of reports emanating from federal agencies, highlighting the so-called crisis, and without the continuing debate in Congress.

More concretely, however, the federal role in Illinois medical education can be seen by examining the amount of money institutions received from the federal treasury. Table 6.2 provides an accounting of the degree of Bureau of Health Manpower support each Illinois medical school received and the purposes for which the money was granted. During the periof of FY 1965 to FY 1975, Illinois schools together garnered $76,874,907, or 4.6 percent of total BHM expenditures for medical education.

It was observed in chapters 3 and 4 that, considering the way health manpower legislation has been written, the major means by which federal monies could be distributed compatibly with state planning would be through the grant review process. Since the administrative decentralization of HEW, the regional offices have had the main responsibility for directing the announcements of grant programs, preparation and dissemination of application materials, assisting institutions with their grant requests, obtaining the services of experts to review the applications, summarizing and rating the applications, and organizing site visits when necessary. The National Advisory Council in Washington and the central HEW administration, however, still had the power to set general policy on criteria for selecting among qualified applicants, as well as final decisions on which institutions would receive the awards.

The HEW regional office responsible for Illinois was ill-prepared to take these tasks on suddenly even under the direction of an experienced member of the central administration transferred from Washington. The combination of new tasks and procedures, new personnel, and understaffing did not contribute to a strengthening of ties to local decision-makers, nor did it greatly improve the federal understanding of local decision-makers or the federal understanding of local problems, both of which were part of the rationale for decentralization. It appears that the regional HEW operations staff has continued to operate under a heavy work load and the strictures of less than optimum communication with the central office.[52]

Despite these limitations, upon reviewing HEW staff summaries and comments, site-visit reports, and other materials pertaining to the major medical education projects funded by the federal government in Illinois, one can detect some effort to consider state planning activity in conjunction with other factors in arriving at a determination of whether or not to recommend approving a project. For the most part, however, acknowledgment of Illinois' master-planning served the purpose of adding credibility to an institution's application by demonstrating that the request for federal money was part of a well-planned, systematic design for the state. There is little indication that federal reviewers ever

Table 6.2. Bureau of Health Manpower Support to Illinois Medical Schools

School	*Formula Grants*	*Special Project Grants*	*Student Loans*	*Scholarships*	*Construction Awards*	*Start-up Grants*	*Teacher Training Grants*	*Total*
Chicago Medical School	3,440,636	2,393,678	613,983	352,450				$ 6,800,747
Loyola University, Stritch School of Medicine	4,910,219	3,873,902	1,749,454	531,114	7,964,973			$19,029,662
Northwestern University	6,093,522	1,914,622	2,539,884	665,622				$11,213,650
Rush Medical College	1,964,823	173,239	309,425	91,838	6,758,080			$ 9,297,405
Southern Illinois University	696,138	87,417	73,516	15,009		2,154,010		$ 3,026,090
University of Chicago	3,829,938	1,558,821	1,449,260	378,340				$ 7,216,359
University of Illinois	10,084,377	5,499,227	2,682,646	948,689	721,669		334,386	$20,270,994
								$76,854,907

Source: U.S., Department of Health, Education, and Welfare, Health Resources Administration, Bureau of Health Manpower, *Selected Information on Health Professions Schools, Part II: BHM Support by Program, FY: 1965-75* (Bethesda, Md.), pp. 27-33.

denied a grant request because it was contrary to the spirit of the Campbell Report; although it should be noted that few in the state would be likely to refute the "more is better" dictum.

Perhaps the clearest illustration of the indirect federal state interaction by way of the grant-review process can be seen in Southern Illinois University's pursuit of a $2,447,616 health professions start-up grant during 1972. SIU claimed that this start-up assistance would enable them to produce an additional 66 graduates by 1977-78. The school argued that with the funds the Legislature had appropriated ($1,971,220 for FY 1972 and $2,412,388 for FY 1973) instruction could begin on schedule, and the $16 million capital development program would continue, but with federal help more students could be trained in a shorter time.

Those reviewing SIU's grant request were operating under the guideline that "start-up funds are not intended to provide the major operating support for the School of Medicine, nor to supplant state funds." Such a determination, of course, is not a simple one for outsiders to make. When consulted, the Board of Higher Education stated that it had encouraged the school to apply for start-up assistance and recognized the impact that these funds would have on future demands, as well as on their own commitment "to recommend such support within limits of available finances."[53]

HEW arranged a site visit for the reviewers who felt they needed a better understanding of the administrative relationships between the Carbondale and Springfield campuses, plans for clinical instruction, the general nature of the curriculum, and more budgetary detail. The site-visit team apparently was satisfied that any concern they might have had in these areas was unfounded, although it is somewhat difficult to discern how outsiders can determine that "no uncertainty or animosity" existed between university and medical school administrators.

Evidently the site-visit team was also impressed with SIU's conformance to the values of the Campbell Report—regionalization of medical education and economy through utilization of existing clinical facilities. Among the supporting documents received by the reviewers was a copy of the Campbell Report, and Dr. Randolph Tucker, research director of the Campbell Report, was on hand during the site visit. Having determined that the state was indeed strongly committed to investing resources in the school and that federal money would not supplant nonfederal funds, the reviewers noted the following, among other points, in justifying their recommendation of approval:

> It was felt that it would be to the detriment of the school if momentum were to be lost at this point in its development through not being able to admit a larger entering class in Carbondale or the class of advanced standing students in Springfield. This is in part related to the necessity to preserve State interest in their efforts, and in part to the need for visibility to prevent loss of State support to other State supported programs in a time of tight money. In essence, this expansion is believed necessary to demonstrate to the State their faith in response to the State's contribution of over $20 million in developmental funds.

There is a need for the community, the State and the faculty to have students on-site as a morale factor, and as visible evidence of progress and productivity by the school.[54]

While it has been generally accepted that federal grants can affect the political balance within a state, seldom is there such an explicit statement of aims as the need to "prevent loss of State support to other State supported programs in a time of tight money."

One key aspect of the review process to keep in mind is that various philosophies abound among reviewers regarding what criteria should be applied in making awards. This has always been clear in terms of the conflicting currents within biomedical research review panels (e.g., whether we would be better off putting all our eggs in the applied-research basket as opposed to that of basic science), but the problem also exists with respect to how one should think about the state effort in relation to federal aid to medical education. For example, contrast the comments of the reviewers involved in the SIU grant request with the comment of one reviewer in the case of a University of Illinois application for construction at Peoria. His remarks are summarized as follows:

The dissenting vote (for disapproval) was based primarily on one reader's opinion that limited Federal construction dollars should not be allocated to the University of Illinois, since State support for capital needs has historically been excellent. Although recognizing that cost effectiveness of the project is reasonable, other alternatives, in his view, including that of State funding in toto, have not been sufficiently explored.[55]

We see here the problem of private federalism as an allocative mechanism. It is usual in a system of competitive grants to value above all factors the quality of the proposal: Is it well conceived and an economical use of funds: Does it have a high likelihood of succeeding in accomplishing the goals set forth?

While there have often been complaints that biomedical research support has not always been distributed equitably among the states, medical education funding by its very nature has this as a major concern. Despite the idea of medical schools as a national resource, the training of physicians has prime significance to states and localities—an important point developed in this case study of Illinois. Is the system that we have been using to disburse federal funds for medical education the most appropriate for overcoming specific health manpower deficiencies?

In theory, the disadvantages of private federalism might be overcome by a system of grant disbursement that is informed about and sensitive to local needs and conditions. One way to achieve this is through strengthened regional offices serving as a conduit in both directions between the local institutions and government agencies and the central office. In practice, this approach—halfheartedly implemented during the early 1970s—has exaggerated some inherent problems in the competitive grant system. The limitations, as identified in a House Committee report, appear to be partially validated by the Illinois experience. It is difficult to secure the requisite manpower, skill, and expertise among regional staff and their consultants to make informed determinations. Common criteria have not always been employed to evaluate similar grant applications. The tendency of local HEW staff and its consultants is to recommend approval of poor-quality applications in order to seek funds for their own regions.

While these complaints could conceivably have been overcome by various types of administrative action, the restiveness of central HEW personnel and Congress itself over lack of control of the award process is not surprising.

With its institutional focus, there was little in the federal program that either encouraged or assisted the states to address health manpower problems in a comprehensive manner. Initiatives were left in the hands of academic institutions to determine their own needs and how they would relate their own imperatives to the needs of their immediate communities and the state as a whole. However, since federal money alone was not sufficient to finance expansion and since states already had commitments for operating support, institutions were obliged to mobilize state action in order to secure matching money and increased operating budgets. In some cases, this forced states to undertake planning activities via legislatures, administrative agencies, or ad hoc commissions, primarily because of critical allocation questions.

In states like Illinois, where the process of reviewing state health manpower goals and overhauling the higher education system had begun, federal funds could be used to fuel a preexisting plan. Federal grants, however, had two major drawbacks. First, because of their competitive nature and the unpredictability of funding, long-range planning in terms of a total state effort was difficult. Second, the changing nature of federal priorities as reflected in the increasing number of strings attached to such broader grants as capitation and the targeting of money for specified purposes (special-project grants) makes coordination with state plans very complicated.

Since Illinois' and federal goals for expansion have for the most part been relatively compatible, the institutions have managed to employ federal funds within the guidelines of the state plans. Whether the medical schools can maintain this mediating role as easily in the future remains to be seen. The reaction to the section of the Health Professions Educational Assistance Act of 1976 conditioning capitation to enrollment of U.S. students in foreign medical schools is perhaps revealing of future federal-state interaction through the medium of medical schools.

In analyzing the impact of this provision shortly after its enactment, the University of Illinois concluded that to accept capitation would cost the state an additional $3.2 to $5.1 million above the current funding base, because the capitation would not cover the full cost of educating these new students. Because so few Illinois residents were in the pool of potential transferees, accepting nonresidents would run counter to the state's goals of increasing medical education opportunities for Illinois residents and increasing the number of physicians practicing in Illinois. Although the federal government ultimately softened its stand on this issue, avoiding confrontation, the University of Illinois' assessment and declaration is interesting from an intergovernmental perspective.

> Because the earlier requirement for capitation, namely enrollment increases, were consonant with the University of Illinois expansion plan and State policy, the acceptance of Federal capitation funds was considered desirable. The new conditions are no longer consistent with those objectives. Accordingly, *the University has chosen not to participate in the program.*[56]

This example represents a relatively straightforward description of the intergovernmental mediating roles medical schools are now called upon to play. The interactional patterns are likely to become more complex as health manpower issues become intertwined with other issues, such as hospital-bed closings, reimbursement reform, and health planning. In the midst of coping with these broad issues, states will be pressing for greater economy in the use of operating funds, local governments will demand continued if not greater service involvement, and the federal government will attempt to pare down its broad educational support but not necessarily lower its expectations of the medical school's role in meeting health-system needs through manipulation of the training function.

Although medical school officials may publicly lament being buffeted by these cross-currents, there appears to be little chance of a return to the past. By building in the capacity to cope with the outside world and by enlarging their scope of influence, academic medical centers have guaranteed a continuing internal pressure for involvement in governmental and social affairs. The growing cadre of personnel who devote their time to policy-making and coordination within the academic health center, as well as liaison to governmental and nongovernmental bodies, will be a major source for this pressure. The linkages that these officials nurture will be seen as a key to the financial ability and often the prestige of the institution. Despite nostalgia for the days of self-contained medical schools, there is growing recognition that deep involvement in the local, state, and national health scene is unavoidable. Medical schools are quickly learning that to stay aloof from surrounding events—the unexpected closing of a municipal hospital, altered state Medicaid reimbursement policy, federal health-planning guidelines—is to court internal disruptions.

NOTES

1. Lester J. Evans, *The University and Education for the Health Professions—The University of Illinois: A Case Study,* 3 December 1964. See also *From Medical Center to Health Center: An Emerging Concept in a Changing World* (University of Illinois Medical Center Faculty Conference to discuss the Evans report), 22-23 November 1965.

2. See, for example, the remarks of University of Illinois President David D. Henry regarding the unique nature of the university's role in higher education in the State. *Faculty Letter,* University of Illinois, 13 December 1963.

3. *Faculty Letter,* University of Illinois, 20 September 1965.

4. George C. Miller, *State of the College,* University of Illinois, College of Medicine, January 1974, pp. 1-4.
5. Ibid., p. 6.
6. Ibid., p. 9.
7. Ibid., pp. 32-33.
8. Rockford School of Medicine, "Program and Philosophy Statement for Community Health Centers for Ambulatory Teaching," Rockford, Illinois, 7 August 1973, p. 3.
9. University of Illinois at the Medical Center, *Campus Report,* August 1972.
10. Rockford School of Medicine, "An Experiment in Health Care and Health Education," Rockford, Illinois, n.d.
11. University of Illinois at the Medical Center, *Campus Report,* August 1972.
12. Rockford *Register-Star,* Illinois, 3 December 1974.
13. Ibid., 16 February 1975.
14. Belvidere *Republican,* Illinois, 21 February 1975.
15. University of Illinois at the Medical Center, *Medical Center News,* March 1976.
16. Rockford *Register-Republic,* Illinois, 18 March 1975.
17. Casey Rice, "The Rockford Story," *The New Physician* 24 (September 1975): 28.
18. Rockford Register-Republic, Illinois, 18 March 1975.
19. Peoria *Journal Star,* Illinois, 9 September 1974.
20. Ibid., 1 February 1970.
21. *Peoria School of Medicine News,* April 1971.
22. Peoria *Journal Star,* 20 October 1972.
23. Ibid., 23 April 1971; 28 April 1971.
24. Ibid., 12 November 1973.
25. Ibid., 11 October 1973.
26. Ibid., 13 October 1973.
27. Ibid., 22 November 1973.
28. University of Illinois at the Medical Center, Office of Public Information, "U. of I. Program to Ease Health Manpower Needs" (press release), 10 October 1972.
29. Illinois Area Health Education System, *Annual Report: Year 03, November 1, 1974 to October 31, 1975,* University of Illinois, College of Medicine, Chicago, p. 53.
30. Ibid., p. 49.
31. Ibid.; see also *Annual Report: Year 01,* p. 32, and *Annual Report: Year 02,* p. 43.
32. *Annual Report: Year 02,* p. 44.
33. Ray E. Wakely, et al., *Number, Distribution and Age of Physicians in Southern Illinois,* Southern Illinois University Area Services Bulletin No. 4, Carbondale, September 1964, p. 18.
34. Michael M. Davis, *Medical Care for Tomorrow* (New York: Harper and Brothers, 1955), p. 412.
35. Joint AMA-AAMC statements released on 5 March 1968 and 16 April 1968. Stevens, *American Medicine,* pp. 374-75.
36. *Innovations in Medical Education: The Springfield Conference,* ed. Homer M. Kimmich (Carbondale: Southern Illinois University Press, 1971), p. vi.
37. Southern Illinois University School of Medicine, "Program Analysis," May 1974, p. 1.
38. Ibid., p. 2.
39. Ibid. (exhibit II), pp. 1-2.
40. Ibid., p. 3.
41. Ibid. (exhibit V), p. 3.
42. "The Assembly on University Goals and Governance," *Daedulus* (Winter 1975), p. 325.
43. Illinois, *Education in the Health Fields* 1, pp. 14-15.
44. Ibid., pp. 24-25.
45. U.S., Department of Health, Education, and Welfare, Health Resources Administration, Bureau of Health Manpower, *Selected Information on Health Professions Schools, Part II: BHM Support by Program, FY: 1965-75* (Bethesda, Md.), pp. 27-33.
46. "Mount Sinai College of Medicine Symposium on Costs of Medical Education," New York, 12 January 1974, p. 34.
47. Chicago *Tribune,* 21 April 1975.
48. Chicago *Tribune,* 15 April 1974, and 18 April 1974.
49. James T. McGill, "An Analysis of a State Program to Increase Physician Retention," *Inquiry* 13 (December 1976): 417-20.

50. James A. Dei Rossi, "Physician Location Choice and State Policy: A Case Study," *Inquiry* 12 (September 1975): 268-70; also, see his reply to McGill, *Inquiry* 13 (December 1976): 421-22.

51. Illinois, *Master Plan,* March 1976, p. 72.

52. Interview with Dr. Robert Hendrickson, Program Officer, D.H.E.W. Region V, 19 April 1976.

53. U.S. Department of Health, Education, and Welfare, unpublished data.

54. Ibid.

55. Ibid.

56. University of Illinois at the Medical Center, College of Medicine, "Statement Regarding Federal Capitation Funds," 19 October 1977.

7

The Varieties of State Action in the Context of the Federal Role

A major problem in the study of federalism is to move from the specifics of a case study describing the relationship of one state and the federal government to generalizations about the national experience. There is always the suspicion that the particular state chosen for study might be grossly atypical. Furthermore, the specific policy area (medical education in this case) may even be challenged as a unique issue that does not shed light on the broad problems of intergovernmental relations.

Unfortunately, there is no completely satisfactory solution to this issue. While for some, the statistical manipulation of quantifiable variables may be a desirable approach, it can readily be seen that much of the data presented in previous chapters does not lend itself to such techniques. And, even if time and resources permitted, fifty more chapters like the preceding one would not necessarily yield valid generalizations about private federalism. In the first instance, we would lose most of what is gained by a case study—richness of detail and an appreciation for the dynamics of policy-making—and in the second, there would be an overload of information.

What is needed is a compromise: The key themes or variables from the Illinois case study must be isolated so that we may see how states might differ according to the types of planning undertaken, the results of that planning, and their relationship with the federal government. In the sense that this study is exploratory in nature, the prime goal has been to understand what the key variables might be and how they might possibly relate to one another. A further step beyond the scope of this study would be to test these emerging relationships to determine the degree of variation among the states.

The design of intergovernmental programs is always complicated by the fact that conditions among states vary enormously. In many programs involving the allocation of federal funds to the states, a wide range of characteristics can be accommodated through the use of formulas, taking into account such objective measures as per capita income, unemployment, and tax effort. In the absence of even these relatively crude measures of state needs, qualitative analysis, the variety of state conditions, and responses in a program designed on the private federalism model is a key to assessing the impact of such legislation.

While it is not the objective of this study to advance elaborate systems models, the categories of "inputs," "conversion," and "outputs" provide a useful means of organizing a discussion of state variation.

INPUTS

Inputs are basically environmental factors that stimulate support and demands for various policy actions. In a proposed research design for a comparative study of health systems agencies, David Falcone identifies four types of inputs: (1) socioeconomic (e.g., measures of urbanism, per capita income, geographic size, ethnic distribution); (2) health service needs and demands (e.g., morbidity, mortality, age structure, utilization); (3) political culture (e.g., political participation, interest-group activity); and (4) medical care system (e.g., health personnel/population, numbers and types of hospitals).[1]

Many of these measures comprising a socioeconomic profile of a state were among the kinds of data that Campbell and his associates gathered in their 1968 report. While it is clear that such data as physician/population ratios are heavily relied upon in rationalizing state medical education expansion, it is unclear exactly how such elements as morbidity data or age structure are translated into guides for state action. Thus, while many health-service need and demand measures may play an important part in supporting an environment that predisposes political action toward expansion, health planning has not reached a level of sophistication whereby these measures can be carefully weighed. In other words, decision-makers are likely to determine health manpower needs on the basis of how their own state or community compares with other areas on certain factors, regardless of the fact that, in other relevant respects, gross differences exist.

As a clue to state variation, however, physician/population ratios tell us little, for even states like Massachusetts and New York, with favorable ratios, decided to expand their medical education capacity. What is probably more important to consider is a state's ability and willingness to invest in medical education, and that is to a marked degree related to its political culture. We must look at the medical education constituency to determine the nature of interest-group activity and its influence on public policy. Who favors state aid to medical education and how do they press their claims?

There are essentially three sources of demand for aid to medical education: those who train physicians, those who expect to benefit locally by the presence of a medical school, and those who have a stake in increased educational opportunity. The composition of each of these is a conglomeration of many disparate interests.

THE MEDICAL EDUCATION ESTABLISHMENT

The medical education establishment, or those involved in training physicians, can look and behave quite differently from state to state. Illinois presents a highly diverse picture with separate public institutions, private institutions with a local orientation, and private schools that consider themselves "national." The structure of medical education in Illinois reflects a higher education system that is also pluralistic and competitive. How does Illinois compare to other states in this regard?

New York, with its relatively new state university system, established in 1948, found itself in somewhat different circumstances because of the historical preeminence of private medical education. It is not so much that private medical school enrollment in New York is proportionately that much greater than in Illinois, but that New York has had a long tradition of close ties between its influential private schools and state government. This special relationship is less likely to exist where there is a tradition of strong, land-grant public schools, as in the Midwest.

Indiana provides an example of a state with one medical school. Its farsighted dean, Dr. Steven C. Beering, has the reputation for dominating health-care politics in the state. He successfully convinced the General Assembly to forgo the idea of building a new medical school and in its stead helped create the Indiana Statewide Medical Education System. This system features regional centers for training students at hospitals and universities throughout the state. While it is clear that care was taken not to snub key interests within the state—Purdue and Notre Dame, for example—the statutory and practical political edge rests with Indiana University. As was observed in an *American Medical News* story on Indiana's system: "Control of the regional center program is not fragmented. It begins and ends in Indianapolis. Thus, student selection, faculty appointments, curriculum development, and administration of the various centers are under the guidance of the medical school administrators and committees, in general, and Dr. Beering in particular."[2]

Except for Rhode Island, with Brown University, Connecticut was the last state to have as its single medical school a private institution. As a result of this singularity, Yale found itself in an uncomfortable position. By virtue of its need for clinical resources beyond its own walls and the broad community involvement of many of its faculty, the medical school naturally developed a unique presence within the state. However, its cherished position as a prestigious national school could not be allowed to be threatened by too close a relationship with the state, which might someday attempt to interfere in such matters as admissions policies. Thus, although it did not relish the idea of another Connecticut medical school, Yale could not vigorously oppose the University of Connecticut's aspirations for a medical college in the Hartford area. Some Yale trustees and the New Haven *Register* did try to discourage this development.[3]

Finally, some states were without medical schools until recently, and several, like Arizona, built their own. The decision to build a medical school, as in Arizona, often creates intense political battles between major universities vying for the prize of the prestigious medical center.[4] Other states wanting a medical school concluded that they either could not afford it or could not marshall sufficient political support to launch a program. As of 1975, seven states were without medical schools: Alaska, Delaware, Idaho, Maine, Montana, Nevada, and Wyoming.

To summarize, the medical education establishment, in creating demands and support for governmental action, can take many forms. States vary according to the number of schools within their borders, the relative number of private and public institutions, and the manner in which schools are related to government.

It should be pointed out that within the category of "those who train physicians" the *medical education establishment* is actually a part of the larger *higher education establishment*. Within this encompassing group, medical education expansion has not always been viewed favorably. While it is true that universities have sometimes waged desperate battles to win medical schools (e.g., Arizona State University versus the University of Arizona), some members of the academic community have been concerned about the drain on funds. This was one concern in the case of Connecticut. Table 7.1 indicates that these worries were not without a basis in reality.

Table 7.1 Appropriations of State Tax Fund for Annual Operating Expenses for the University of Connecticut, 1970-71 to 1973-74 (in thousands of dollars)

	1970-71	*1971-72*	*1972-72*	*1973-74*
University of Connecticut (nonmedical/dental)	$40,048	$44,700	$44,321	$44,963
Medical/Dental School	9,109	13,191	13,729	15,813
Total	49,157	57,891	58,050	60,776

Source: M. M. Chambers, *Higher Education and State Governments, 1970-1975*, p. 64.

COMMUNITY GROUPS

The expansion of medical education, as was seen with Illinois, is not restricted to the involvement of education and government officials. It is a community affair in the sense that a number of local interests perceive that they will in some way benefit from the presence of a medical school. In general, three types of groups in the community have played key roles.

One such group encompasses those preoccupied primarily with economic development—the business or civic leaders and their partisans in local government. Added to this is an element of boosterism often associated with the development of a new medical school. Sometimes it takes the form of traditional city rivalries, like those between Tucson and Phoenix or between Hartford and New Haven. In other cases, it is a matter of the civic duty that comes with the self-perception of being a civic leader. Invariably, foundations are formed to help finance some of the new facilities or to provide matching money for federal grants. It is not unusual for these committees associated with fund-raising activities to have a part in policy decisions as well.

The actions of the business community can fuel city rivalries, but they can also dampen competition when things get too hot. Merlin K. DuVal, the first dean of Arizona's medical school, has described the reaction to a 1962 report recommending establishing a medical school in Tucson, which resulted in a petition campaign by the citizens of Phoenix:

> Even as signatures were being gathered it became apparent to the business leaders of the two major cities that the harm being inflicted on the state by this quarrel could outstrip the importance of the issue itself. Because of the common concerns shared by the people of both cities in public utilities, branch banking, water, and other natural resources, it was decided therefore that a single dramatic step should be taken to bring the initiative petition to a halt.[5]

By the time the legislature was ready to meet to appropriate the necessary funds, the issue, which they would have had to settle (or would have been unable to settle), was politically defused.

Perhaps even greater controversy has been engendered not in *which* city a medical school is located, but in *what part* of town it should be built. The problems of San Antonio are reminiscent of the debates surrounding the selection site for the Peoria Medical School:

> Controversy over the site continued, and in April 1961 the Downtown Merchants and Property Owners Association appeared before the regents and urged that a downtown location be chosen for the new medical school. Land in an urban renewal area was selected by the group, but the Urban Renewal Agency could not guarantee that the land would be available for construction immediately. The group favored the downtown site because of already existing medical facilities in the area and closer proximity to a large indigent population. Location of the school in that area would facilitate surrounding property development and promote interest in the central business district.[6]

Unlike Peoria, the business community of San Antonio was unsuccessful in winning its case.

Of course, demand for medical school expansion does not solely derive from the business community, but from the general public as well. It is difficult, however, to pin down exactly how this demand is communicated. Suffice it to say that legislators generally believe that their constituents are concerned about doctor shortages, and in varying degrees of sophistication they connect solutions to this problem with aid to medical education. Actually, a state legislator is usually so deeply rooted in his constituency by virtue of his many organizational memberships, lifetime residency, and shared ethnic and religious affiliations that he needs little direct prompting or encouragement about the issues that will please the voters.[7] Considering the number of towns and ghetto areas without doctors and the attention that the press has given to the "doctor shortage," it is not surprising that the building of new medical schools is about as important an accomplishment as any to point to in answer to the political question: "What have you done for us lately?"

In addition to the business community, general public, and medical education establishment, there is another influential force operating for expansion. This is composed of those who deliver local health-care services.

While it has often been assumed that organized medicine opposed the increased production of medical graduates and did its best to discourage expansion, the activities of state and local medical societies do not support this assessment—at least during the 1960s. In many instances, medical societies helped to spearhead the drive for new medical schools. That is not to say that these moves were taken without some trepidation, however. While advantages could be gained by the presence of a medical school in terms of continuing education, the opportunity for part-time teaching positions, and improved facilities and services for one's patients, there were disadvantages too. There were the potential put-downs by snobbish academic physicians, as well as possible interference in the affairs of local hospitals by medical school administrators. And, no doubt, the possibilities of intensified economic competition could not be disregarded.

In Illinois, the State Medical Society, responding to a 1971 State Senate Resolution requesting them "to recommend to the General Assembly the best means by which this state can interest physicians to decentralize their practices by making themselves available throughout the state," endorsed the state plan for regionalization and medical school expansion. The society emphasized the importance of a physician's free choice in practice location and urged that attempts to deal with geographical distribution rely on improved incentives to attract new physicians. To this end, the society was strongly supportive of such mechanisms as community preceptorships and loans with forgiveness clauses.[8]

In some states, the medical societies went beyond endorsements and cooperation to active lobbying. Just prior to the 1968 elections, the Texas Medical Association filed statements with the Texas Republican and Democratic platform committees urging them to support aid for both the expansion of the existing schools and the creation of two new schools. The association pointed to the widening gap in physician/population ratios and the poor comparative position of the state with respect to the rest of the country (Texas 1 M.D./997 persons; U.S. average 1 M.D./681). It noted the need for more family practitioners and physicians in rural areas. And, interestingly, it offered the observation—and one that is no doubt particularly disturbing to a Texan—that "only 45 percent of the physicians who have joined the Texas Medical Association since 1961 are natives of Texas."[9]

To take another example, the California Medical Association has described its position on aid to medical education:

> CMA's commitment to an adequate supply of health manpower to meet California's future needs is underscored by our active campaign on behalf of Proposition One in 1970, which failed, and Proposition Two on the November, 1972 ballot, which voters approved. CMA contributed staff and financial assistance toward the passage of these bond issues to upgrade and expand the state's medical schools and other health manpower training facilities.[10]

Even though the Ohio Medical Association is considered by some to be one of the more conservative groups in organized medicine, it has a history of vigorous support for state aid to medical education. For example, the Ohio State Medical Association House of Delegates passed a resolution in 1967 advocating the construction of additional medical schools in the state. When Governor John Gilligan's 1973 task force recommended that new medical schools not be established, the medical society stood by its original resolution.[11]

Along with varying degrees of pressure from organized medicine, the community hospital sector has also viewed medical education expansion favorably and has gladly added its support. Here was the chance to upgrade equipment and expand physical plants through medical school affiliations that would bring increased state and federal aid. Here was the promise of attracting a high-quality staff and graduate medical education programs.

The increased use of community hospitals was at the heart of many state plans for medical education expansion. Cost effectiveness, regionalization, and the orientation of medical students to community practice were the goals. Yet, while some parts of the academic community were attracted by a new age of experimentation in medical education, others remained skeptical. Compromises were often rationalized on the basis of "the price one has to pay" in order to find necessary funds. Attempts to put together coalitions of groups with different priorities often resulted in conflict.

The planning of a medical school at the University of California in San Diego provides a telling illustration. Campus officials in San Diego had one idea of the type of institution that should be built: "The new San Diego School of Medicine was not to be a great medical school from the outset, dedicated to the training of physician-scientists. It could only accomplish this from a solid campus base."[12] To carry out the philosophy, a teaching hospital on the campus would be essential. But community forces had different ideas, which included a county hospital-based medical school. The obvious and eventual compromise, the use of both a campus and a county hospital site, was reached in a larger historical and political context:

> The university [the University of California System] and the legislature had both been appalled by what they regarded as the unreasonable escalation during the fifties of the size and cost of the UCLA medical school. Motivated primarily by the desire to increase the output of practicing physicians, legislative leaders were suspicious that the university would produce "another research institute" in San Diego. University officials, feeling the hot legislative breath on their neck, bore down hard—especially since they were aware that the campus had no intention of creating a "diploma mill."[13]

As we have seen, the demand for government expenditures in the area of medical education springs from a number of sources within the community. The general public and the professional public, in the form of local hospitals and organized medicine, have in their own fashion lent support to increased spending. Having looked at those who train physicians and those who expect to benefit from the training enterprise, our attention turns to a third group—those who are primarily concerned about educational opportunity.

PRESSURE FOR INCREASED EDUCATIONAL OPPORTUNITY

In essence, the third group is an artificial construct, for it can easily be considered part of the general public. Analytically, however, the distinction is useful, for the nature of this group's demands are somewhat different in that the improved organization and delivery of health-care services is an indirect goal subordinated to the goal of providing more spaces in the state's medical schools. Within the general clamor for increased opportunity to get into medical school, the voices of minority groups have been heard and to some extent heeded.

While it would be difficult to measure the comparative policy impact of this type of pressure from state to state, there is a general impression that both middle-class and minority pressure have on occasion made their mark. New York, for example, is often cited as an example of a state in which middle-class pressure on the legislature has been particularly intense. This was not always so, however, for in one of its earlier reports, the state's concern was over "the stiff competition for qualified youth offered by other remunerative and prestigious professions and sciences."[14] The situation was to change soon thereafter as medical school places became highly sought-after.

It is not unusual for states to stress in policy documents the importance of providing greater opportunity for state residents. Indeed, it is sometimes a convenient rationale for expansion in states with comparatively favorable ratios. The general pattern is to deplore the indignity of being a "debtor" or "predator" state leaning on less well-endowed states. It is also common to deplore the fact that residents must seek their education in foreign countries with questionable medical education standards. And, finally, there is the medical-schools-are-a-national-resource argument. Maryland, for example, provided a rather elaborate discourse on its "responsibility to meet the Nation's Physician Needs":

> The dilemmas posed by any attempt to project future needs in a given state, based upon all the variables, are wiped out once one removes the blinders created by state lines. When one recognizes that we are all part of one nation, and that medical education is essentially a national problem, not a state problem, then a single index of need is practicable. The index, of course, is the accepted physician/population ratio projected to determine the *national* need for physicians. if we meet the national need in terms of quantity of physicians, then by proper distribution we can meet population needs in all areas of the nation.[15]

CONVERTING DEMAND INTO GOVERNMENT ACTION

While the nature of demands and supports vary among states, so too does the functioning of governmental institutions for processing these demands. A reasonable question to ask is whether this variation makes much difference in the kinds of policies produced in the successful implementation of those policies. Although a definitive answer to this question is beyond the scope of this study, we can take the first steps to try to determine in what ways political institutions vary and to hypothesize about possible effects.

The key institutions to consider are the governor and his staff, the legislature, and the major, responsible state agency. The prime task for analysis is to identify the locus of power among these actors and determine basic patterns of political interaction between interest groups and government officials.

In Illinois, the governor and legislature played only a minor role in the expansion of medical education beyond that of accepting the Illinois Board of Higher Education's master planning recommendation on the manner of expansion and the pricetag associated with it. While determining how large a slice of the budget pie a social service like higher education deserves is no small matter, in the case of Illinois, legislative and gubernatorial participation was minimal. Once a sense of how much money the state can afford was gained, the board and the educational institutions were relatively free to hammer out a plan and to follow it. The question of whether the board had real power or was merely the captive of the educational institutions is not easy to answer, since no serious tests of will developed. On those occasions, however, where threats to harmony arose, the board appeared to handle the situation adroitly. The board's power has to date been well demonstrated in the realm of what Robert O. Berdahl calls "the de facto exercise of 'nonpowers.'" "The Illinois coordinating board," he says, "was granted the power to make only budget recommendations; but since its recommendations were always accepted virtually intact by the state government, the institutions soon began to take this fact into account, and any evaluation of board powers should recognize the psychological reality."[16]

Does this same pattern of converting demands for medical education expansion into governmental action prevail in other states? The following mini-case studies have been chosen from the literature to illustrate the variety of patterns that seem to have been present during the late 1960s and early 1970s.

Illinois' neighbor Michigan has had a long tradition of institutional autonomy in which higher-education interests have managed to resist the incursions of the legislature and administrative agencies. In this context, the Michigan medical education story, as told by John Walsh in *Science*, provides an interesting contrast to Illinois.[17] The major political battles in Michigan seem to be fought primarily in the legislature. Walsh describes the general process:

> The legislature's leverage in dealing with medical schools is exerted, not surprisingly, through the power of the purse, and the fulcrum is the appropriations committees of the state senate and house. But the mechanism that sets Michigan apart from other states is a joint capital outlay committee. This is a six-member body—three from the senate, three from the house—which examines proposals for new state-funded capital construction and makes recommendations which are almost always accepted by the legislature.[18]

The work of this committee is characterized by its long and numerous meetings, its competent staff, and the flexibility to employ the service of outside consulting firms.

One of the cardinal issues this committee had to face over the years was whether to approve the establishment of a medical school at Michigan State University. Recalling the reasons for opposition to this venture, MSU's dean, Andrew D. Hunt, listed the obstacles the medical school's proponents encountered:

> 1. The medical schools of the University of Michigan and Wayne State University needed funding for their commitments to expand medical education and felt that these commitments should be met before any new program was established at MSU.
> 2. Michigan State had grown too fast and was exceeding its mandate by moving into the field of medicine; such an effort would be unlikely to succeed in a "cow college."
> 3. Clinical resources in the Lansing area were quite possibly inadequate to support a full medical program; Detroit or Grand Rapids would be more appropriate sites for a third medical school when such an institution was called for.
> 4. Even though a 1962 resolution of the Michigan legislature permitted MSU to proceed with a "two-year program in human biology leading to the M.D. degree," it was the general feeling that the university was planning for a college without appropriate mandate from the body politic.[19]

An interesting twist in the Michigan story was provided by the state's osteopaths, who at the time were estimated to have made up to 17 percent of the total supply of physicians in the state and one-third of the general practitioners. Although fully licensed and recognized by organized medicine, this cohesive group tends to be hypersensitive about second-class medical status. However, apparently they were quite popular in the legislature, partly because they have been perceived as dedicated to rural, primary-care practice in contrast to their colleagues. When the osteopathic lobby decided to seek funds for support of an osteopathic school, the legislature, in what Walsh describes as "a shotgun wedding with the legislature holding the shotgun," decided that it would be more economical to join the osteopathic school and a new medical school under one roof—Michigan State University.[20]

While the legislature could probably not have withstood MSU's pressure for a four-year school indefinitely, the school was established only at a cost of numerous compromises imposed by the lawmakers, who have influenced the character and operation of the school.

There has been some continuing interest on the part of the legislature and governors in devising a formal system of accountability. The Appropriations Committee, in 1972, engaged the services of the firm of KMB Health Systems Inc. with the idea of obtaining a better fix on costs in relation to program effort. The medical school deans did not particularly relish the idea of program budgeting with its burdensome requirements for defining programs in detail, categorizing expenses, identifying revenue sources, and linking both income and expenditures to particular programs. While the deans balked at first, they eventually relented and have generally cooperated with KMB.[21] As M. M. Chambers commented on these developments in Michigan:

> Most state budget directors are coming to admit that the mandatory conversion can be accomplished only after years of "shaking down," and that there is serious question as to whether any beneficial outcomes will result, even if the thing can be done. No one seems to ask whether it is needed or is likely to be worth its huge cost in added administrative and clerical work, and in the depressed morale. It is the fad of the times since the days of McNamara and his "whiz-kids" in the Defense Department, and a few more years may elapse before it peters out and gives way to the next cost-accountant's fantasy.[22]

Program budgeting in the McNamara sense has not been instituted per se as far as Michigan medical education is concerned. The KMB study was completed in 1976. The medical schools cooperated, although certain pieces of information were just too difficult to provide. Michigan budget officials feel they will be able to make some use of the study even if it has not proved to supply the kind of answers one needs in order to make tough allocative decisions.

Our analysis of Michigan, a state with strong legislative leadership, should be tempered with a look at North Carolina. The statutory powers of the governor are exceedingly modest. Meanwhile, the newly formed higher-education coordinating mechanism, the Board of Governors, was only beginning to make its presence felt politically when a major controversy over a new medical school arose. Thus the legislature was to play a key role.

The legislators in the eastern section of the state—a group that tends to dominate legislative committees through its seniority—have long been interested in securing a public medical school for their region, the existing medical schools being located in the central and western sections. As early as 1965, the legislature authorized a medical education program at East Carolina University. By 1972, a one-year program was instituted at East Carolina in cooperation with the University of North Carolina at Chapel Hill. Two years later, the General Assembly suddenly decided to change the *Statewide Plan for the Expansion of Medical Education* that the Board of Governors had previously submitted. In their Appropriations Act, the legislature outlined:

> The Board of Governors of the University of North Carolina is hereby directed to submit to the General Assembly in its operating budgets for the 1975–76 fiscal year comprehensive plans (1) to expand as soon as practicable the program of first-year medical education at the East Carolina University School of Medicine, and (2) that concentration be placed upon the training of family care physicians, and (3) that special efforts be taken to encourage the recruitment and medical education of racial minorities.
>
> In carrying out the purposes of this Act, the University of North Carolina School of Medicine at Chapel Hill and the East Carolina University School of Medicine shall work cooperatively toward full accreditation of the expanded medical education program at East Carolina University to the end that its graduates may transfer freely to other units of the University of North Carolina School of Medicine.[23]

To support this plan, a sum of $15 million was appropriated.

The North Carolina developments are complex and interesting from a number of perspectives. We will return to this case to illustrate other points later in this chapter, but meanwhile the role of the legislature in the affair should be reviewed in the present context. Despite the vociferous opposition of North Carolina medical education leaders—a group that consists of many nationally respected and influential educators—and despite the opposition of the university president and against the better judgment of the Board of Governors, the legislature was able to force the state university system to design and operate a medical school that its leaders did not want. However, one might interpret the attitudes of medical education leaders as another example of seeking to maintain the status quo. Also, given the progressive nature of U.N.C.'s leadership and interest in new forms of health-care delivery, special credence is lent to the view that the legislative role here was dysfunctional, suggestive more of pork-barreling than of rational planning in the public interest.

Having examined instances in which the state legislature has been the key to important decisions regarding medical education, our attention now turns to a case in which a governor has dominated the decision-making process.

In his study of higher-education politics in New Jersey, Richard Halverson relates an interesting account of Governor William Cahill's 1970 efforts to merge Rutgers Medical School and the New Jersey College of Medicine and Dentistry. The latter school was a private four-year institution that went public in 1965. Rutgers, a two-year state-supported school, had aspirations of becoming an academic medical center. The governor, however, was convinced that Rutgers was heading in the wrong direction—toward research rather than toward an emphasis on the production of primary-care practitioners. He also believed that a more effective use of state resources could be achieved through a merger. According to Halverson: "All respondents agreed that the merger initiative was the governor's own and that he acted without stimulation from other political leaders or interest groups." Reportedly, Republican legislators were willing to support the governor "because of long-standing animosity between them and the president of Rutgers, who had been closely associated with Democratic politicians during the 1960's." Rutgers could not successfully marshal support from either other New Jersey colleges and universities or the Board of Higher Education, which made no formal recommendation of the proposal. Rutgers' major support emanated primarily from a group of state doctors and the president of the Association of American Medical Colleges. But this was not enough; the governor prevailed.[24]

Indiana represents a state that departs from the patterns previously discussed by virtue of a tradition in which decision-making is delegated for the most part to academic institutions. Chambers characterizes the Indiana situation:

> Well-known for many years for amicable and efficient allocation of state resources among the several public institutions of higher education, and progressive development of the statewide system by means of voluntary coordination, involving continuing careful fiscal collaboration by the staffs of the four principal universities, but wholly without any statutory structure or officious state bureaucracy for higher education, Indiana was the last domino to fall in the unstoppable collapse toward statutory "coordinating boards." In 1971 the legislature, having only two years earlier rejected out of hand a proposal for an all-powerful single governing board, established a mild type of "soft-approach" coordinating board styled in the Indiana Commission for Higher Education.[25]

In the realm of medical education, the dean of Indiana University has been given considerable statutory power, greater perhaps than any other medical school dean. The dean is ex-officio member and chairman of a medical education board, the purpose of which is to direct the Statewide Medical Education System.[26] The significance of this development is not that the dean has become the state's medical education dictator, but that the focus of the political activity has been displaced from the governmental sector to the quasi-governmental university sector, with the medical school dean playing a key role.

The four major types of political interaction patterns in which demands for medical education are translated into governmental action have been examined. In Illinois, the focal point was an administrative agency, in New Jersey the governor, in Michigan and North Carolina the legislature, and in Indiana the higher-education institutions themselves. A fifth category can probably be discerned in which power has either traditionally been fragmented or in which power has shifted from one part of the decision-making structure to another.

Although they barely acknowledge the fact, the states, the federal government, and voluntary sectors, each within its own sphere of policy-making, influence one another's decisions in the area of medical education expansion. As was seen in the previous chapter, the federal government intentionally and unintentionally made its presence felt in several respects as the states and their medical schools attempted to formulate and implement expansion plans. While it was not overtly a key factor in Illinois, the accrediting powers of the voluntary associations can also have an effect on the direction of state planning.

The state's dilemma with respect to these two external forces has been addressed, if not solved, by the authors of the Wisconsin Governor's Health Planning and Policy Task Force. In their final report, they noted the "lack of organized knowledge regarding the programs and plans of the many health professions schools. Even the plans of the major public systems such as the University of Wisconsin or the vocational and technical system are not subject to orderly coordination and planning for rational use of the state funds," they complained.[27]

A further look at attempts to establish the medical school at East Carolina University will help clarify the measures by which voluntary associations may act as external forces influencing state policies. The construction of a new public medical school in a state is always a sensitive affair. The established school[s] will attempt to head off the development either by voluntarily decentralizing or attempting to scuttle the plans of the interloper.

In North Carolina, an interesting twist was provided by the actions of the Liaison Committee on Medical Education, the joint accrediting body of the AMA and AAMC, when it virtually forced a cooperative agreement between UNC and East Carolina. Neither UNC, East Carolina, the Board of Governors, nor the General Assembly had originally anticipated or sought the kind of formal agreement that eventually resulted. UNC, for example, had planned either to expand its own facilities at Chapel Hill or to form an arrangement with North Carolina State University in nearby Raleigh. The LCME, however, would not accredit East Carolina as a freestanding, two-year medical school unless it came under the auspices of the UNC, with assurances that Chapel Hill would maintain a sufficient degree of control over admission, promotions, curriculum, and faculty at East Carolina.[28]

Before concluding this section on external forces, something should be said concerning the role of private philanthropy. While the proportion of private resources in medical education financing has diminished over the years, there are occasions in which private individuals and organizations have greatly influenced the planning process. Needless to say, foundations like Carnegie and Josiah Macy have had their impact via their many general reports on medical education. The Commonwealth Fund and others were instrumental, especially in the 1960s, when interested state groups needed planning grants to investigate the feasibility of new medical schools. Finally, there is the considerable impact of the large private donation, as exemplified by the medical school of Pennsylvania State University, which owes its existence chiefly to the Milton Hershey Medical Center trust. The dean of that school, George

T. Harrell, provides an edifying account of some of the political problems associated with a medical school so founded:

> All direct contact with the state government and the legislature is made by central university administration. Key members of the legislature expressed concern that they had not been involved in the original decisions setting up the medical school. The nature of the trust fund and the negotiation with the governor and court leading to the original allocation precluded easy involvement of legislators. This concern has been expressed repeatedly in committee hearings on budget requests in subsequent years.[29]

OUTPUTS AND OUTCOMES

As we have seen, states vary according to the nature of demand for medical education and with respect to the locus of decision-making power within the governmental structure. It is beyond the scope of this study to relate on a national scale variation to variation in structure on outputs and outcomes.

If one simply views the desired outcomes of state policies (outputs) to be the expansion of medical education, then, in most instances, state governments were fairly successful in achieving their target enrollments. The more complex and illusive goal of improving access to health services for state residents through manpower policies is much more difficult to measure and will probably require the passage of several years, by which time the practice patterns of recent medical graduates will have been established.

In the interim, however, it is appropriate to pose a few pertinent questions about state policies that may in future help in the assessment of the quality of state actions, especially in the context of the federal role.

Do states try to plan for their physician needs, or is the supply merely the result of a conglomeration of ad hoc decisions, incremental budgeting actions, and individual institutional planning?

Obviously the answer to this question depends on what one calls "planning." All planning, to a certain extent, involves ad hoc decisions, incremental budgeting actions, and individual planning. However, semantics aside, the important issue to reconcile is whether state governments have the capacity to cope with basic social issues. In the area of health manpower, we should be concerned about what kind of job state policy-makers have done in assessing the state physician-supply needs and how they have acted upon those assessments. There is little ground for dismay over the federal government bypassing the states, unless the states have demonstrated some capacity or interest in the problem of maintaining an appropriate physician supply.

Given the brief synopsis of state efforts in this chapter and the detailed analysis of Illinois, it is apparent, however, that states do plan. To be sure, the sophistication and governmental apparatus for planning varies among states. The reason for expanding the supply, the fiscal resources for undertaking expansion, and the means to monitor constantly the implementation of an expansion also varies. But states do plan.

Did states perceive their physician supply problems at the same time and in the same manner as the federal government?

There is little evidence to suggest that either the federal government or the states can be given sole credit for setting in motion the "doctor shortage" bandwagon and the subsequent medical education expansion. If anything, they were mutually reinforcing. Medical educators and administrators with schools in financial difficulty appealed to *both* federal and state policy-makers. Rural and inner-city voters complained to state legislators, mayors, governors, U.S. congressmen, and the President. While some states may have begun their expansion prior to the first federal intervention, there is no telling how far and fast they would have proceeded without a strong federal role. However, federal intervention was influenced by subtle encouragement from the states.

If state authorities plan, do they do so rationally or are they overwhelmed by powerful interest groups? Are they able to implement their plans efficiently and economically? Do the plans work?

Incontestably, the face of U.S. medical education has changed considerably since the early 1960s. We have more institutions, more students, and a whole set of new relationships between the major participants in the medical education sector. Many of these changes result from decisions made by state authorities. Were these decisions fair? Did they make sense? Were they in the public interest? Were the goals achievable and worth achieving?

To begin with, one must accept the premise that state policy-makers—or any policy-maker—cannot be expected to transcend the best available knowledge and advice. While some are beginning to question the decision to expand as vigorously as the nation did, there were few who outspokenly opposed those moves in the 1960s. Few policy decisions are ever based on the overwhelming weight of the data, but many are based on the overwhelming appeal of an idea at a particular moment in history. And so it was with expanding the physician supply.

Given the tenor of the time, some states seem to have been able to pursue the goals of improving the size and character of their physician supply with more success than others. Continuity of leadership is probably the key factor in predicting success.

In Illinois, continuity of leadership was provided by the Illinois Board of Higher Education. Although its leadership and membership changed over the years, the board was a dependable forum that was capable of designing, implementing, and monitoring a plan. Despite the expected disagreements over particular decisions, few would argue that its mode of operation was unfair or arbitrary.

Michigan, it would appear, also developed continuity via the legislature. However, the legislative committee described by John Walsh would seem to be a unique development in comparison to most state legislative committees.

In general, a state higher-education coordinating board might be the best hope for establishing and maintaining continuity of leadership. Legislatures, through their appropriation powers, will never be completely out of the game; however, in most cases, substantive committees do not have the resources or inclination to do the kind of detailed work required.

A governor wishing to have a significant part in the planning process must rely on his budget bureau or some advisory mechanism, either an individual adviser or an ad hoc commission. Like legislators, governors will always have some say in the planning process through their various powers, but can they provide continuity of leadership through advisory mechanisms that by definition lack continuity?

If we are to make any distinctions between states that are more or less successful, then we will have to settle for answers to the following questions:

1. How explicit were state planners in framing their goals in the first place? Were state plans a prescription of logical steps to follow in achieving goals, or were they merely pious statements about the need for more doctors?
2. Were goals realistic in terms of the state's ability to finance them? For example, was the contingency of a federal diminution of effort taken into consideration?
3. Did planners take into account factors that might impinge on the realization of goals? A delicate balance must be achieved between including key interest groups, communities, and government agencies in the decision-making process and allowing the planning process to be captured by any one group.
4. Is it made clear who is responsible for overseeing the implementation of the plan? Do the overseers have evaluation capability to determine whether goals are being achieved, and do they have enough flexibility to adapt to changing conditions and new perceptions?
5. Ultimately, we must ask what has been accomplished and at what price? But we should pose these questions with the understanding that it is an unrealistic expectation to believe that complex social systems can be swiftly changed. It is not so much whether we have failed or succeeded, but how much of a dent we have made in the problem.

What part, if any, do local communities play in state planning?

The study of intergovernmental relations involves not only federal-state relations, but the relationship between these two entities and local communities. Because local governments do not finance medical schools the way they do community colleges, for example, there has been a common misconception of the part that communities have played in the history of medical education.

As we have seen, local community groups and governmental agencies have been key sources of demand for medical education. In the implementation phase, communities have been involved in decisions concerning use of county and city hospitals, the location of medical school buildings, and the fund-raising efforts of community groups. Perhaps most interesting has been the growing involvement of communities in what some would call the internal affairs of the medical school. This trend, a consequence of medical school decentralization in the pursuit of solutions to the geographic maldistribution problem, is one that deserves further attention in the years to come.

Do federal funds add to state planning efforts? Or do they frustrate them? Or do they not make much difference?

Addressing the 1975 National Governors' Conference, Governor Phillip W. Noel of Rhode Island made some observations that are particularly pertinent to a discussion of the federal influence on state planning.

> I know I have testified on behalf of the Governors before the Senate and the House of Representatives on health planning and regulation legislation as it was emerging in Congress, and I got the distinct feeling that the people in Congress didn't trust the state government. They didn't think that Governors had the capability of dealing with such a vital area of service. That's my own opinion, but I got that sense, that attitude, when I testified before the Congress of the United States.
>
> I sit here today and hear Governors say or indicate that they don't have a sense of trust and confidence in county executives and mayors. I think that's what is wrong with all of the domestic programs in the country. The President, the Congress, state government, local government, county government, we don't have a system where one level truly trusts the other and, if we don't trust each other, then we are not going to be able to work cooperatively. Whether it is state-local finance or health planning and health delivery systems, we all are in the same business and we all represent the same people. Governors have to trust the county executives and county executives have to trust mayors and Congress has to establish a new understanding and recognize that local government and state government have capabilities.[30]

To say there should be more trust among levels of government may seem obvious and not particularly constructive. Nevertheless, upon closer inspection, the governor's observations do get at the heart of the problem of private federalism.

The tacit assumption in private federalism is that federal aid to medical schools is a matter that does not concern the state; it is a private transaction between the federal government and the medical schools. It is also implied that the states do not have the capability to manage the normal intergovernmental method of a pass-through of funds, as, for example, in the Hill-Burton program, where states are given jurisdiction over disbursement of funds to private hospitals.

Of course, federal policy-makers did not consciously choose private federalism over normal intergovernmental patterns. As we saw in the chapters on the federal role, private federalism is more or less a product of the historical relationship of the federal government to medical schools with respect to research funding. While the issue of whether this was an appropriate way to fund medical education was raised in the beginning by a few members of Congress whose responsibilities centered more on education than on health, it was quickly dismissed as an unimportant concern by the legislation's sponsors, who were of the congressional health committees.

We will never know what might have been had the federal government organized its intervention in medical education in the normal scheme of federalism. Certainly, decisions regarding hospital construction have not all been wise ones. So there is no assurance that the states, in complete control, would have necessarily done a better job of planning.

How, then, might we deal with the question of whether private federalism was a dysfunctional way of structuring the federal role? The evidence from Illinois and other states reviewed does not seem to suggest that the federal role grossly distorted state planning efforts. There are few examples of outright confrontation between a state and the federal government over funds made available to a particular medical school. There are few instances of major crises in which medical schools have defied state planning because federal funding gave them an independent power base.

NOTES

1. David Falcone, "The Challenge of Comparative Health Policy for Political Science," *Journal of Health Politics, Policy and Law* 1 (Summer 1976): 207-8.
2. American Medical Association, *American Medical News*, 1 October 1973.
3. John W. Patterson, "University of Connecticut School of Medicine," in *Case Histories of Ten New Medical Schools*, eds., Vernon W. Lippard and Elizabeth Purcell (New York: Josiah Macy, Jr., Foundation, 1972), p. 122.
4. Merlin K. DuVal, "University of Arizona College of Medicine," in Lippard and Purcell, *Case Histories*, pp. 1-32.
5. Ibid., pp. 5-6.
6. F. C. Pannill, "The University of Texas Medical School at San Antonio," in Lippard and Purcell, *Case Histories*, pp. 1-32.
7. Thomas R. Dye, *Politics in States and Communities* (Englewood Cliffs, N.J.: Prentice-Hall, 1969), p. 140.
8. Illinois State Medical Society, "Response to Senate Resolution No. 119," 20 October 1971.
9. "Statement Filed with Political Parties," *Texas Medicine* 64 (October 1968): 113.
10. "Health Manpower," *California Medicine: The Western Journal of Medicine* 6 (December 1973): 53.
11. William R. Schultz and Peter Lancione, "Minority Report to the Report of the Governor's Task Force on Health," *Ohio State Medical Journal* (March 1974).
12. Clifford Grobstein, "University of California, San Diego School of Medicine," in Lippard and Purcell, *Case Histories*, p. 92.
13. Ibid., p. 98.
14. New York, State Committee on Medical Education, *Education for the Health Professions*, June 1963.
15. Maryland State Planning Commission, Committee on Medical Care, *Medical Education and Research Needs in Maryland: Report of the Subcommittee on Medical Education and Research*, January 1962, p. 18.
16. Robert O. Berdahl, *Statewide Coordination of Higher Education* (Washington, D.C.: American Council on Education, 1971), p. 25.
17. John Walsh, "Medicine at Michigan State (I): Educators and Legislators," *Science*, 22 September 1972, pp. 1085-87; "Medicine at Michigan State (II): The Architecture of Accountability," *Science*, 6 October 1972, pp. 36-39; "Medicine at Michigan State (III): Conditioning for Innovation," *Science*, 20 October 1972, pp. 288-91.
18. Walsh, "Educators and Legislators," 22 September 1972, p. 1087.
19. Andrew D. Hunt, "Michigan State University College of Human Medicine," in Lippard and Purcell, *Case Histories*, p. 174.

20. Walsh, "Educators and Legislators," 22 September 1972, p. 1087.

21. Walsh, "Architecture of Accountability," 6 October 1972, pp. 37-39.

22. M. M. Chambers, *Higher Education and State Governments, 1970-1975* (Danville, Ill.: The Interstate, 1974), p. 135.

23. University of North Carolina, Board of Governors, "The Expansion of the East Carolina University School of Medicine: Recommendations of the President to the Committee on Educational Planning, Policies, and Programs and the Committee on Budget and Finance," 8 November 1974, p. 2.

24. Richard Field Halverson, "Institutional Influence in the Politics of Higher Education in New Jersey," (Ph.D. diss., Columbia University, 1975), pp. 246-51.

25. Chambers, *Higher Education*, p. 96.

26. Steven C. Beering, et al., "Statewide Medical Education in Indiana," in U.S., Congress, House, Committee on Interstate and Foreign Commerce, *National Health Policy and Health Resources Development: Hearings Before the Subcommittee on Public Health and Environment*, 93d Cong., 2d sess., 1974, pp. 334-39.

27. Wisconsin, *Final Report of the Wisconsin Governor's Health Planning and Policy Task Force*, November 1972, pp. 83-84.

28. University of North Carolina, Board of Governors, "Report of the Committee to Study the Request of East Carolina University for a Second Year of Medical Education," 29 December 1972, pp. 9-19.

29. George T. Harrell, "The Pennsylvania State University, The Milton Hershey Medical Center," in Lippard and Purcell, *Case Histories*, p. 364.

30. *Proceedings of the National Governors' Conference*, Washington, D.C., 8-11 June 1975, pp. 108-9.

8

Conclusion

Regardless of whether one's predilection is for massive reform of the American health-care system, designing new programs to satisfy unmet health-care needs, or for simply making the present programs operate more effectively, there are two questions ultimately to be confronted when governmental action is contemplated. How should responsibility be shared among the levels of government? What functions should the private sector perform?

Partly, contradictions are due to the nature of policy-making in a democratic society, in which, as Herman Somers points out, the lack of coherence is not unique to health care. "Where controversy is many-faceted and deeply felt," he notes, "the only way to a unified and consistent national policy is through authoritarianism."[1]

Part of the explanation also lies in the nature of American federalism. The founding fathers provided no recipes for intergovernmental action. The power dynamics are evolutionary, "ground out of experience," in the words of Richard Leach, who further observed:

> Although both the national government and the states have ample power under the Constitution on which to base action, there is no clear statement or implication therein to guide either as to when or how to exert it, either singly or in combination . . . nor is there any guidance to the private sector as to when or how it should act.[2]

Prior to direct federal and state efforts to address physician shortages by expanding medical education capacity, a fragmented system of private authority governing physician production had evolved. In response to both internal pressures for a more coordinated approach toward medical education and growing government interest in the performance of private groups carrying out "public" functions, the medical education sector is beginning to demonstrate some capacity for self-evaluation and cohesiveness in dealing with government. Despite persistent suspicions that private authority has contributed unfairly to restricting the levels of medical school output, government programs to expand the supply have continued to work through the present system, dominated by private authority rather than by a more strictly managed public system.

Private medical schools have always reserved the right to determine for themselves when and how to expand, while the academic leadership in public medical schools has demanded an important voice in these matters. Hospitals have decided the size and types of residency programs offered. Accrediting agencies have influenced guidelines for expansion in the name of preserving quality. This is not to say that government has totally abrogated its authority in designing and administering its incentive programs. Indeed, the precarious financial position of medical education institutions and the fragmentation of responsibility within the private sector itself has permitted governments a certain freedom to drive recipients of aid in directions they might be reluctant to go.

States have had a traditional role in supporting public medical education. However, the 1960s saw major new initiatives with respect not only to increased financing for expansion but for more purposeful planning. The impetus for this planning was something that pervaded all of higher education—a belief that the educational system ought to be more closely linked to the social needs of the state. This linkage could only be accomplished by establishing objectives, assessing current resources, and developing a system of higher education. Characteristically, this involved efforts to overcome geographical inequities in the distribution of institutions, provide greater opportunity for minorities, create a more effective administrative apparatus, and bring private institutions into the mainstream of state planning through grant programs.

The federal program was essentially modeled on the relationship that developed between the federal government and medical schools with respect to biomedical research funding. This private federalism applied to the area of health professions education and excluded the states from direct involvement in the design and administration of the federal health manpower program. Interaction between states and federal authorities was, for the most part, indirect through the medium of the medical schools. Yet, because states were expected to help provide matching monies and, in the case of public schools, to maintain the expanded enrollments through increased operating support, their stake in the federal program was quite high.

After little more than twelve years following the first infusion of federal funds aimed specifically at expanding health professions education, there has been scant evidence of either much cooperation or conflict between the federal and state governments. It cannot be said that the federal program during this period interfered greatly in the capacity of states to shape and manage their own expansion programs. Potential problems have been avoided for two basic reasons. First, there was a general consensus that more money to produce more doctors almost anywhere was a good thing—or at least not a harmful thing. Second, the medical schools became adept at putting together state and federal funds, minimizing conflict between the two levels of government.

This unstated arrangement among the three sets of actors is undoubtedly one that will come under considerable stress in the near future. The assumptions underlying the dramatic push to expand medical school capacity are beginning to be seriously questioned. The potential, deleterious side effects of oversupply are worrying some policy-makers, while the disappointments over the limited impact of an increased supply on reducing costs or providing care to underserved groups are frustrating others. It is within this climate that medical schools will be searching for operating funds to maintain increased enrollments and new programs. Their coordinating role will become increasingly difficult. In attempting to live up to the commitments of the past, they must extract operating funds from a reluctant federal government and financially pressed states, both of whom are not beyond exacting new requirements for what support they give.

THE MEDICAL EDUCATION SECTOR

In assessing the future of the three-cornered relationship among the medical education sector, the federal government, and the states, it is important to take into account both the benefits derived by each of the partners from the current arrangement as well as the stresses produced in this largely uncoordinated approach.

Interest groups comprising the medical education sector perform the same functions traditionally ascribed to other political interest groups in the American democratic society: They are shared-attitude groups that make certain claims through or upon government. The preceding chapters contain numerous examples of how groups like the AAMC attempt to obtain favorable decisions for their medical school constituents with respect to governmental aid and other related concerns. As noted throughout the study, the medical education community is highly differentiated. Thus there are groups representing research interests, the specialties, hospital interests, and so forth, and within these groups there is a continual struggle to maintain internal cohesion among a membership that may differ on the basis of regional, functional, or structural characteristics.

Aside from the lobbying function that interest groups perform, there is another side to the policy arena that seldom figures in American political analysis, but it is nonetheless a significant aspect of medical education politics. Much of the control of the production of physicians is voluntary and government must take on the role of an interest group in lobbying for changes in this voluntary system.

Samuel Beer, relying in part on Eckstein's British Medical Association analysis, describes how producer groups can exercise sanctions by virtue of "the denial (in various degrees) of advice, acquiescence, and approval—which can cause, to put it mildly, 'administrative difficulties' and which, by anticipation, endow the group with bargaining power in its relations with government." Beer explains: "The source of this power is not the fact that the group or its members has a role—for instance, as voters or contributors to party funds—in the system of parliamentary representation, but derives from the group's performance of a productive function."[3]

Although the analogy with Britain should not be stretched too far, the comparison is instructive in providing perspective on evolving organizational arrangements in U.S. medical education politics. The formation of the Coordinating Council on Medical Education is a response to the need to establish an instrument for negotiation between the voluntary governing structure and the federal government. The critical development to watch in the coming years will be the shifting relations among the associations represented on the CCME as that body attempts to satisfy government's need for a cohesive producer group with which to negotiate.

The effectiveness of the CCME will be greatly dependent on its ability to voice the broad concerns of the medical education sector without representing the parochial interests of the parent associations. The search for a workable modus operandi has lead the CCME to consider such issues as the approval process for reports, the financing and hiring of staff, and the appropriate relationship to the federal government with respect to controlling graduate medical education.

If an acceptable and convincing organizational posture could be achieved, the CCME could contribute considerably to health manpower policy decisions. This would be particularly the case where standard setting is an issue, such as in specialty mix, reimbursement, shortage areas, and licensure. Given the unlikelihood that we will ever be able to provide definitive answers to these complicated questions through research alone, some degree of consensus within the medical education community would be of immeasurable assistance—especially if Congress continues to demand greater control over the health system.

Comparable developments can be seen also at the state level. When state governments took on the task of addressing physician-supply problems, they quickly realized that the academic medical center was inhabited by different interests. State officials needed a negotiation agent from the medical center—someone to provide information about where to apply funds and someone to be held accountable for the use of those funds.

The extent to which interest groups in Illinois were given a direct voice in the formulation and administration of policies to expand the physician supply suggests a functioning negotiation model. In this respect, the development and implementation of the Campbell Report was more than a matter of interest groups merely influencing government officials or being taken into account, but an assumption on their part of a formal role in planning, budgeting, and administration. It is important to realize that the government did not abdicate its responsibility; such an abrogation of responsibility would preclude negotiation. Rather, one sees a cooperative effort characterized by bargaining.

As explained in Chapter 7, a variety of conditions prevails from state to state relative to the numbers and kinds of medical schools and their relationship to governmental institutions. However, some general points about the continuing role of medical schools in state policy-making can be stated.

The fragmented system of financing medical education has enabled each medical school, based on its own resources and institutional goals, to put together a budgetary package by relying on several different sources to varying degrees. For example, a research-intensive school pursues different funding options than a more locally oriented school. Despite the propensity of medical school deans to describe their condition with the tired metaphor of marching to the beat of different drummers, there is a certain flexibility in the system that does not exist in many other countries with more stable financing.

With the advantages of this lack of strict accountability to a single funding source, certain disadvantages are also apparent. The financial outlook for medical schools is a curious mixture of contradictions that will continue to plague their administrators. In order to maximize revenues, medical schools have had to extend their scope of influence and expand their organizational capacity to deal with the various funding sources. In some ways, this has strengthened their internal cohesiveness because more money was available for central administrators to control, and it became clear that government agencies needed a negotiating agent from the institution. However, although expansion produced a heightened awareness of the importance of coordinated management, the reality is that medical centers are indeed more complex now and are that much more difficult to oversee.

Inherent in the structure of academic medical centers is the uneasy union among three major power centers—the university, the medical school, and the teaching hospital. The forces driving these components do not always produce a solid front to government, as illustrated in the following comments by the president of a large university system:

> There is a very real possibility in a time of constrained resources that medical schools will become a drain on the rest of the university. It is tremendously important that they not do so, for, as I have stated earlier, they are a vital part of the university but also dependent on work done in other disciplines within the university. There is an understandable temptation, especially when funds are scarce, to seek special funding for medical schools. Faculty in the schools have access to important segments of the public in ways faculties in other parts of the university do not. They must be careful not to abuse that access.[4]

The stresses are also apparent in the relationship of the hospital to the university and medical school. The former dean of Harvard Medical School suggests one viewpoint commonly held in the medical education community:

> The present organization of medical education allows neither the university nor the teaching hospital to fulfill its proper role. Perhaps a first step might be to recognize that the teaching hospital is not now, and cannot be, an integral part of the university and that attempts to force the teaching hospital into this mold are damaging both to the university and to the hospital. The recognition that the university and the teaching hospital are equal but separate institutions would facilitate their relations with one another with the government and with the public in the years to come.[5]

Adding to these organizational tensions are two other related interests. One potential faction is the group of community hospitals and other facilities now commonly in the medical school orbit. Another consideration that has received little treatment is the interrelationship of the other health professional schools and the medical schools. Nursing deans in particular have balked at any sign of medical school domination. Yet, it is possible that in the tradition of such programs as AHEC, cooperative efforts among the health professions schools within a university will be necessitated.

Finally, in states with several medical schools, the political picture is complicated by the potential for competition for limited state resources, as well as for cooperation in addressing health manpower and service needs on a regional basis. Both tendencies have been exhibited in the past. While there have been several examples of two state universities vying for support to build a new medical school or well-established medical schools discouraging the development of potential competitors, the higher-education community in general banded together to generate increased medical school appropriations. The extent to which medical schools will be required to apply political pressure in the state budgetary process for continued operating support or further growth is dependent, at least in part, on local economic conditions, public enthusiasm, and the degree to which the state appropriations machinery either encourages or minimizes inter-medical-school rivalries.

THE FEDERAL ROLE

In the Health Professions Educational Assistance Act of 1976, Congress declared: "Health professions personnel are a national health resource and the Federal Government shares the responsibility of assuring that such qualified personnel are available to meet the health care needs of the American people." The often-repeated declaration that health manpower is a national resource has served as a useful shorthand statement of the rationale for federal involvement in physician and other health professions training. The rationale was based on the recognition that medical schools were unevenly distributed among the states. Physicians are a highly mobile professional group. With its investment in research, entitlement, and hospital construction, the federal government had some interest in assuring that a sufficient supply of health personnel was available and that educational institutions not succumb as a result of serious financial pressures.

Acknowledgment of health manpower and training institutions as a national resource only established the appropriateness of a federal role in addressing the goals listed above. It does not automatically confer entitlement to a specified share of the U.S. Treasury, because there are other items of national importance also with claims on the limited tax dollar. A retrospective view of federal health manpower legislation and executive action since 1963 reveals a series of limited measures and financing experiments—construction, financial distress, a variety of loan and scholarship programs, targeted special projects—rather than a long-term commitment. The closest Congress has come to such a commitment is capitation, an unpredictable program that federal policy-makers are continually attempting to phase out.

The inability of the federal government to make a long-term financing commitment to medical education is linked to a second major unresolved issue. Despite the sentiments expressed in the 1976 health manpower legislation concerning the fact that the federal government "shares the responsibility" of assuring the availability of health professions personnel, too little attention has been paid to the manner in which that responsibility has been shared with the states. Seldom does one see any direct acknowledgment of a state role in federal legislation, hearings, committee reports, or public statements, let alone an attempt to determine the response or impact of federal funds on state goals and activities as in most other programs.

It should be recognized that stable, consistent operating support of institutions through direct grants is not what the federal government does best. The federal government is good at focusing attention on problems, getting everyone excited about solving those problems, deliberating on alternative solutions, marshaling its data resources to define the global parameters of the problem, and inciting others to action. The federal government should learn to use the levers at its disposal more proficiently. Medicare and Medicaid reimbursement policies represent one such lever with potential for effectiving positive changes.

Another limitation of the federal government is that it cannot do the kinds of planning that state governments can and often do. Despite numerous reorganizations and attempts to decentralize HEW for the purpose of bringing the government closer to the people, the task of learning about complex institutions like medical schools and their relationship to other parts of the health-care system in a state is beyond the capacity of federal officials whether they be in the regional offices or in Washington. The federal grant-review process is simply too ad hoc. With its reliance on outside consultants and overextended bureaucrats, it is an ineffective way of determining whether a new project will work or whether a new institution is needed within a particular environment.

Although state governments suffer limitations, the opportunities created by various routine state activities—budgeting, legislative appropriations, capital development, planning, and statistical reporting—add to the likelihood that a more realistic and feasible approach to health manpower can be managed at the state level rather than at the federal level.

None of this means that the federal government has no place in financing and shaping medical education. On the contrary, the federal government does have a role, but this role must involve maximizing what it does best and minimizing functions it does less well. In other words, federal officials should continue to investigate problems from their national vantage points, mobilize public interest and support, and experiment with manipulating the large flows of money from the federal treasury. These are areas in which states are weaker. Yet, the valuable tools and expertise at the disposal of the federal government are virtually useless to the states if deployed in almost complete ignorance of state policy and planning.

THE STATE ROLE

At the state level, medical schools exist in the two policy realms of health and higher education. Both have experienced rapid expansion in past years, and concomitantly state government has become increasingly interested in coordination, regulation, and planning.

In higher education, all but three states had by 1974 established some kind of coordinating agency. While educational specialists debate the extent to which these coordinating boards are able to wield genuine power, compared to health planning agencies they are notably more stable and influential. Herbert Klarman lays some of the blame for the ineffectiveness of health planning efforts at the door of the federal government:

> It is my opinion local health planning in this country has been hindered by the federal government in several ways. One is obvious, namely the unreliability and instability of funding for health planning that is inherent in project grants. The latter make for concentration of effort on getting money and for discontinuity of substantive activity. Too, there has been an ebb and flow of federal funds—sometimes they are on the rise, sometimes they are on a declining trend, and sometimes they are being redeployed. One effect has been to displace existing agencies with experience before the new planning agencies have taken hold and matured. Experience, which often is the accumulation of knowledge on what not to do, is wasted.[6]

Although the National Health Planning and Resource Development Act of 1974 mandates manpower planning as one responsibility of the local health systems agencies, whether manpower and facilities planning will come together remains to be seen. Even while Congress was simultaneously deliberating on separate health planning and health manpower legislation, neither bill was seriously discussed in the other's hearings—despite the fact that the bills were considered by the same committees. At one point in the House health planning hearings, Congressman Paul Rogers had the following exchange with Frank C. Carlucci, HEW Under Secretary:

Mr. Rogers: Who plans for manpower, local?

Mr. Carlucci: That is a local level function, but you would have a statewide coordinating council that would integrate the plans.

Mr. Rogers: Do they overrule the local group, the Statewide? I thought you said the State would not overrule.

Mr. Carlucci: This is essentially a coordinating council. They would not overrule the local groups.

Mr. Rogers: Then what happens if the local group says, "We need 20 surgeons, 200 nurses and 140 dental technicians," and so forth? What do they do about it?

. . . .

Mr. Secretary, what I am concerned with is, I am not sure that you can really do all of the manpower planning from this local base. It has to be Statewide for a State. For the national, it has to be national. I presume you would agree with that?

Mr. Carlucci: Yes, sir. to the degree the States are running, or funding, health manpower training, obviously, they have an important role. But they should seek, in our judgment, and will seek, the advice of local health systems agencies in terms of what their assessment is of the local manpower needs. I don't think we need to mandate by Federal statute a coordinating mechanism to have that happen. I think this will happen naturally.[7]

It seems then that for the next few years physician supply planning at the state level will continue to be part of the budget and review process for higher education. As discussed in Chapter 7, this is not always solely under the purview of higher-education coordinating agencies in each state. Yet, even where other parts of state government play a role in decision-making, the context is usually the higher-education budget, although the rhetoric may be "meeting the state's health needs."

Given this context in which political decisions regarding medical education are likely to be made, general developments bear close watching:

1. What effect will budgetary problems experienced by university systems have on their medical schools? There are several possible variations on this theme. At one extreme, strong university presidents may be able to make tough allocative decisions reducing the medical school's share of the total pie as the university's share is reduced. In other cases, medical school budgeting may be more independent of overall university budgeting. However, the consequences of a medical school with its own sizable income—whether from a separate endowment, research overhead, or patient-care services—may result in resentment from other parts of the university.

2. It will be interesting to watch for second thoughts about new or expanded medical schools. There has already been such talk of medical schools that should never have been built. Reports about the demise of medical schools at the University of California in Irvine[8] and the University of Massachusetts,[9] for example, were numerous in 1975. Yet, however much these institutions might be judged to be a drain on state fiscal resources, the political resources necessary to close a medical school are perhaps even greater. The real test may come in states without the resources of California or Massachusetts. These poorer states lack the budgetary flexibility to recover from the ebb and flow of federal funds. They are finding themselves paying the bills for the care and feeding of facilities built with federal dollars. If the idea ever takes hold that we may have trained too many doctors, public officials may be less likely to fear taking a hard line on budgetary matters where once sacrosanct medical schools are concerned.

3. While both the states and the federal government are beginning to pursue more aggressive policies aimed at ameliorating geographic and specialty maldistribution, it is conceivable that differing views by the two levels of government over what is accountable behavior on the part of the medical schools may lead to conflict. Since private federalism militates against the state and federal government working out their differences, the medical schools in the middle will do their best to appear to be complying with both.

4. The role of local government and local interest groups in the development of policy for an expanding physician supply is greater than previously acknowledged. Local political actors have involved themselves in pressuring state officials to increase medical school places, in the location and construction of new medical schools and health-care facilities, and even in the internal personnel struggles of the medical school. Whether the health systems agencies (HSAs) mandated by the 1976 planning legislation will accelerate attempts to influence physician supply planning from the local level is difficult to say at this early juncture. Nevertheless, local decision-makers will no doubt have some budgetary influence so long as medical education continues on the track of community service and local elites sit on higher-education boards and commissions.

5. While many states have adopted the principle of public aid to private medical education, the future is an uncertain one. State subsidies have increased from $7,599,000 in 1965–66 to $74,059,000 in 1974–75, growing from 0.9 percent of total medical school support to 2.5 percent.[10] For many schools and states, this aid is problematic.

Prior to federal health professions support, private schools in serious financial trouble faced either oblivion or the prospect of turning public. For example, three of the schools in the State University of New York system experienced the latter fate. While this is less of a prospect in the 1970s than it was a decade or two earlier, private schools are obliged to reconcile the temptation of state subsidies with a potential loss of autonomy, which is far short of going public, yet disturbing nonetheless. As for the state, the problem is to come to terms with an appropriate mechanism of accountability for private institutions.

PRIVATE FEDERALISM: A FIRST ASSESSMENT

The American health-care system is pluralistic and its power is fragmented. Many notions about health-care reform start from this point, and consequently we search for the incentives that will move the pieces of the system in the directions we think are right. When this fails, our efforts turn to regulation—pushing the pieces rather than coaxing them.

When officials at all levels of government began to worry about an inadequate physician supply, they first designed incentives to encourage medical schools to expand and to encourage students to choose medicine as a career. While not everyone in the medical education establishment was convinced that new schools ought to be built and old ones expanded, they were convinced that medical schools' financial position required new support from the federal government as well as more support from the state. The medical schools and the students responded well to the incentives.

Governmental intervention has essentially been incremental so that, although problems such as geographic maldistribution were recognized early, few efforts to meet the problems directly were attempted. Much faith was placed on the judicious location of new medical schools, the utilization of community hospitals, the provision of educational experiences in primary-care settings, and programs of recruitment to bolster the supply of minority and rural physicians.

If there is any truth to the constantly repeated dictum that it takes at least ten years for a new medical school to go from the drawing board to graduating its first class, then certainly there has not been adequate time to assess the effects of these programs, most of which were not begun until the late 1960s and early 1970s. Yet, Congress and several states apparently feel that more direct measures are required. And this undoubtedly has as much to do with the growing sense of confidence among policy-makers that government has a rightful place in the affairs of the medical education sector as it has to do with any real knowledge about the impact of past initiatives or the likely effects of new incentives that verge on regulation.

Federal, state, and local governments each pursued the broad objective of expanding medical education capacity. Each, however, also works within its own frame of reference. From the federal vantage point, the disparities between New York and Mississippi, between urban and rural, between "have" and "have-not" schools, are what come to the fore on a national scale. State officials are primarily concerned with intrastate disparities, allocating higher-education resources among competing institutions and providing greater educational opportunity. Local communities are also concerned with these issues, but they see the presence of a medical school in terms of increased medical services and economic development.

In view of these similar goals but different perspectives, what evidence is there to indicate that the mechanism of private federalism is dysfunctional in terms of state/local activities? In the absence of open conflict, one must consider the possibility that states were encouraged to pursue ineffective policies or that the federal program's design prevented a potentially constructive working relationship among the levels of government.

Although "doctor shortage" skeptics may rightly dispute the cost benefits of our large investment in physician-supply expansion, there is little reason to believe that a different form of intergovernmental relations would have persuaded policy-makers to respond differently to the conventional wisdom of calling for more doctors and more medical schools. Nonetheless, one wonders whether some of the positive features of direct intergovernmental transfers that exist in other programs may not have also benefitted our health manpower efforts.

The equalizing effect among the states of hospital facilities, for example, was a major accomplishment of the Hill-Burton program. The program, which allotted funds to states on a formula basis ensuing an intitial grant to a state-designated agency for surveying and planning hospital needs, was said to have had the following impact:

> The simple relationship between number of beds per capita and state personal income per capita that was so strikingly positive in the early forties disappeared; indeed, the reverse is now true for short-term hospitals. The Hill-Burton program was a factor in achieving these goals.[11]

While caution is required in comparing the expansion of hospital resources to human resources, one is struck by the more direct attack on the problem of hospital maldistribution in contrast to the basic approach chosen for manpower distribution. Perhaps joint federal-state cooperation might have provided greater opportunity for considering a more judicious use of funds.

Another important benefit accruing from the traditional intergovernmental relationship is a strengthening of state capabilities to deal with problems. Martha Derthick, in her study of federal influence in the area of public welfare, found that federal initiatives aided in the professionalization of state bureaucracies.[12] Similarly, a study of the impact of federal child-health programs on the state of Connecticut demonstrated that despite a number of deficiencies, such programs can have a marked impact on improving the administrative capacity of state bureaucracies.[13]

Robert Connery, et al., in a study of the Community Mental Health and Retardation Act, concluded that one cannot avoid the reality that states are "the crucial building blocks of the federal system" and suggest that the federal role must be a flexible one taking into account disparities among state capacity and administrative structures.[14] Thus if state agencies are weak, then the federal government should assist in strengthening them—bargaining with the governor's office if need be to ensure a strong agency or applying pressure on the states by fostering local interest. It is most important that the states retain their role as full partners in the implementation of the program, and in turn the federal program will benefit from the state agencies' detailed knowledge of real problems.

Together, state and federal funds greatly increased the output of the nation's medical schools. Private federalism cannot be faulted for hampering this effort. Yet, it must be remembered that increased supply was not an end in itself but a means of improving access to health-care services. There remains considerable skepticism over whether there has been enough progress toward this goal to justify the large public expenditures. Even the anticipated secondary benefits of securing a more stable financial base for medical education and increasing medical education opportunities for minorities has not been fully realized.

POLICY DIRECTIONS

If one had to characterize the distinctions between the mid-1960s and mid-1970s in terms of health-care developments, it would probably be fair to say that there has been a shift from concern with extensive resource development—both manpower and facilities—to the predominant themes of cost containment, rechanneling of resources, regionalization, and integration of facilities planning with manpower planning. These mid- and late 1970s themes are far from new, but they take on a different cast under circumstances of constraint.

As difficult as it was to eradicate the failures of the health-care system during an era of massive growth, it will be that much more of an elusive goal now.

With this cautionary note in mind, I will conclude this study by identifying three related issues that are likely to be influential in shaping the health manpower agenda in the next several years. These are issues that require reformulation. In particular, it will necessitate reorienting our thinking with respect to the manner in which the federal government ought to relate to the states.

The first issue involves the interrelationship among various types of health manpower. The interplay of political and economic forces that link the fate of physicians, nurses, and allied health groups in the future of the American health system was beyond the scope of this study. However, there is much in the experience of these groups that parallels the expansion and transformation of the physician supply as a response to state and federal policies. So long as there was a perceived critical physician shortage by policy-makers at both levels of government, there was little impetus to examine some of the underlying assumptions about the integration of the various professions and the long-run economic implications.

Although the term *substitution* has been used extensively by health manpower planners, the extent to which and the manner in which "new health practitioners" substitute for physicians in practice is yet to be fully understood. Notwithstanding the potential of such personnel to provide high-quality care, which has been well demonstrated, there are some important open questions about their wide-scale use. In particular, concerns have been voiced regarding levels of productivity and inefficient deployment.

However, it has been argued that new health practitioners exist not solely to substitute for physicians but to satisfy unmet needs in the sense of services that physicians for the most part have lacked interest in delivering. This often refers to much of what comes under the rubric of preventive services. The degree to which services are significantly expanded is dependent on a host of public policy factors, not the least of which involves difficult reimbursement decisions.

An additional side to the question of manpower mix involves another relatively unexplored concept—competition, both within individual health professions and among professional groups. In their justifiable zeal to explain why the classical competitive market does not apply to health field, health economists have neglected to delve deeply into other aspects of the concept of competition. The focus has primarily rested on the nature of competition with respect to overall costs and the medical profession as a whole vis a vis the consumer.

Competition may underlie a good deal of political activity in the future. It would be improbable to expect wide-scale unemployment or a serious decline in physician incomes. Nonetheless, the behavior of interest groups with respect to the politics of reimbursement, licensure, and government regulation may very well reflect a concern with competition.

In addition to the matter of manpower interrelationships, there will be increasing attention paid to ways of improving the linkages between manpower programs and facilities planning. The beginnings of a conscious attempt along these lines can be seen in the implementation of three federal programs—AHEC, the National Health Service Corps, and the Health Resources Development and Planning Act.

The concept of the Area Health Education Center by its nature is an embodiment of the conjoint goals of developing manpower resources and expanding services in scarcity areas. In the absence of extensive objective evaluation of the program, it is difficult to determine the extent to which it represents a substantive departure from usual medical school/clinical services arrangements. The 1976 legislation in principle refines and enlarges the program. It is expected that inner-city areas will be represented in this expanded effort.

The National Health Service Corps is another program that, like AHEC, has in its early, limited stages begun to test the capacity of the federal government to link service delivery and manpower training. The stipulations concerning site development prior to the assignment of corps personnel have required some creativity on the part of a federal bureaucracy, which often functionally separates service delivery and manpower training. At present, the National Health Service Corps remains an experimental program, at least until Congress reinforces its expressed intent in the 1976 Act with sustained increases in appropriations.

Finally, opportunities are presented by the planning legislation of PL93-641. In the past, federal health planning legislation has been synonymous with facilities planning. Some analysts, Rosemary Stevens, for example, are pessimistic about the impact of HSAs on issues like manpower distribution in light of their tendency to concentrate on facilities planning. She suggests that primary manpower activities will be "to develop census-type information about manpower in defined health service areas, to identify areas that are underserved with respect to aid under Federal programs, and to provide a forum for discussions of manpower development, and a possible stimulus for change."[15]

While these are not inconsequential tasks, it is uncertain whether they alone will contribute substantially to manpower and facilities coordination. To a great extent, specific progress along these lines will depend, first, on the willingness and ability of HEW to designate approval of health manpower programs in a meaningful way. Second, the willingness and ability of state authorities must be directed toward this goal of coordination. Maryland, for example, has moved to organize relevant health manpower education groups in the state into a council for the purpose of coordinating manpower planning with other HSA activities.[16]

A third broad issue, in addition to interrelationships among different types of health manpower and the integration of manpower and facilities planning, involves the question of the financing of academic medical centers. It must be recognized first that the previous two issues are not unrelated to this third concern. In other words, one cannot reasonably separate developments in other parts of the health system from medical education.

Another important prerequisite for addressing the issue of medical education finances is a recognition that given the structure of medical school revenues it is impossible to insulate these institutions from the currents of health politics. The pursuit of a revenue base unaffected by political pressures is the medical education sector's Eldorado. It is an unrealistic goal and one that if achieved would undoubtedly lead to stultification.

This does not signify that the present situation cannot be improved. To a large degree, medical school financial problems are individualistic, growing out of the economic and political climate within which the institution operates, as well as its history and structure. If a medical school is saddled with an unprofitable teaching hospital, for example, the solution to the problem is not to be found in the magic bullet of federal capitation funds, but in complex negotiations at the community level that may ultimately involve parts of the federal and state bureaucracy. Financial problems of medical schools have many and varied causes, and a variety of sources must be explored for their solution.

The view that financial problems of medical schools are rooted in multiple causes, thus requiring the deft manipulation of several resources can be extended to a general approach toward potential reforms within the intergovernmental context. Namely, no one party among the medical education sector-federal-state/local triad can make much progress in curing the deficiencies of health manpower production and deployment without the cooperation of the others. It is not a question of finding the perfect formula for coordination, devising the single financing mechanism that assigns appropriate fiscal responsibility, or establishing a super-regulatory board. Improvements, rather, are more likely to be achieved through an understanding of how the system operates and through discrete actions aimed at overcoming specific inadequacies in its functioning.

To address in our governmental system concerns like geographic maldistribution—an issue that even countries with more centralized health-care-delivery systems find highly problematic—it will require action directed at the needs and based on the resources of a manageable health service area. Hopefully, such action will be inspired at the local level, more specifically by the health system agency (HSA). However, given the diversity of the U.S.—both in terms of the severity of local problems and the capacity to deal with them—we must expect varying degrees of success. This in turn demands a certain flexibility on the part of federal and state agencies in devising policies that will stimulate the effective use of federal, and state dollars, expertise, and regulatory authority.

As I have attempted to demonstrate, the private federalism of medical education financing evolved as it did in response to a number of political and structural circumstances. It seems questionable whether this mechanism is suited to meet the health manpower challenges of a postexpansionary period where gains will be sought through a more rational integration of resources. If we are to make headway toward this goal, the federal government and the states can no longer rely on indirect communication.

NOTES

1. Herman M. Somers, "Health and Public Policy," *Inquiry* 12 (June 1975): 90.
2. Richard H. Leach, *American Federalism* (New York: W. W. Norton, 1970), p. 61.
3. Samuel H. Beer, *British Politics in the Collectivist Age* (New York: Vintage Books, Random House, 1965), pp. 330-31.
4. David S. Saxon, "Is the Medical School a Proper Part of the University?," *Journal of Medical Education* 51 (December 1976): 995.
5. Robert H. Ebert, "Medical Education in the United States," *Daedalus* 106 (Winter 1977): 183.
6. Herbert E. Klarman, "National Policy and Local Planning for Health Services" (Lecture delivered on the campus of the University of Missouri-Columbia, 21 January 1975), p. 12.
7. U.S., Congress, House, Committee on Interstate and Foreign Commerce, *National Health Policy and Health Resources Development: Hearings Before the Subcommittee on Public Health and Environment,* 93d Cong., 2d sess., 1974, pp. 499-500.
8. Robert Gillette, "Health Education in California: The Grand Design in Trouble," *Science,* 18 April 1975, pp. 239-41.
9. Association of American Medical Colleges, *Weekly Report,* 9 February 1976.
10. Sylvia I. Etzel and John J. Fauser, comps., "Medical Education in the United States 1975-1976," *Journal of the American Medical Association,* 27 December 1976, p. 2970.

11. Judith R. Lave and Lester B. Lave, *The Hospital Construction Act: An Evaluation of the Hill-Burton Program, 1948-1973* (Washington, D.C.: American Enterprise Institute for Public Policy Research, 1974), p. 47.

12. Martha Derthick, *The Influence of Federal Grants* (Cambridge, Mass.: Harvard University Press, 1970), pp. 158-89.

13. Christa Altenstetter and James Warner Bjorkman, "The Rediscovery of Federalism: The Impact of Federal Child Health Programs on Connecticut State Health Policy Formation and Service Delivery," in *Public Policy Making in a Federal System*, eds. Charles O. Jones and Robert D. Thomas (Beverly Hills: Sage Publications, 1976), pp. 217-37.

14. Robert H. Connery, et al., *The Politics of Mental Health: Organizing Community Mental Health in Metropolitan Areas* (New York: Columbia University Press, 1968), pp. 585-86.

15. Rosemary Stevens, "Health Manpower," in *Regionalization and Health Policy*, ed. Eli Ginzberg (Washington, D.C.: GPO, 1977), pp. 107-19.

16. On 10 August 1977, an interagency agreement was signed between the Maryland Comprehensive Health Planning Agency, the Statewide Health Coordinating Council, the State Board for Higher Education, and the State Department of Education (Division of Vocational Technical Education).

Index

About the Author

Michael L. Millman is a research associate on the staff of the Conservation of Human Resources Project, Columbia University. Trained in the disciplines of political science and health services administration, he holds a Ph.D. from Columbia University and a MPH from Yale University. Dr. Millman, editor of *Nursing Personnel and the Changing Health Care System* (1978), has published and lectured in the areas of intergovernmental relations, health manpower, public hospitals, physicians' attitudes, and on the role of municipal governments in the delivery of ambulatory care.